NO JUNK REPS

Every Outcome Is the Correct
Outcome for the Process Applied.

GARY WISE

TESTIMONIALS

I have worked with Gary for nearly 2 years now, and what I am most impressed by is his attention to the smallest details in a person's mind and behavior. He inspires me to be the best version of myself because that is what Gary shows me every day, both physically and mentally.

Le Khanh Hung
University of Illinois Freshman, 2026
Junior Presidents Cup, 2024
Vietnam National Team Member
32nd South-East Asia Games, Individual Champion

In all honesty, Gary Wise is one of the most impactful people I have ever met. Before meeting Gary, I believed in my mental strength. I had never needed to discuss a process with a mental coach until I was introduced to him. Getting to know him was truly a pleasure, and having the opportunity to discuss specific mental topics is always incredibly valuable. Gary explains things in a way unlike anyone I have ever met, and I am genuinely grateful to have someone like him by my side.

Filip Jakubčík
University of Arizona Junior, 2025
European Amateur champion, 2025
2x Western Collegiate champion
The Open Championship participant 2025

I have known Gary for almost 5 years now, and he just never stops impressing me with how much he knows about training minds. He is such a nice person and a great guy to be around. I'm really impressed with how much attention he pays to you when you're working with him and how he notices every little detail that might be holding you back from being the best version of yourself. I'm super grateful to have him as a coach.

Gerardo Gómez
University of Arkansas Sophomore
Mexican National Team
Mexican National Amateur Champion 2024

I've been working with Gary for four years. The most significant improvement has occurred over the past year. In the last six months, I've also grown tremendously as a person thanks to Gary's guidance. He helped me develop mental strength, which I believe is the most crucial and challenging aspect of golf to master. Last year, I faced many struggles in both golf and life, but applying the lessons Gary taught me helped me emerge from my lowest point. Most importantly, I learned a great deal from experiencing setbacks.

TingWei Chang
University of Oregon Sophomore, 2025
26th Faldo Series Europe Grand Final Champion

In my 25 years in the well-being and high-performance world, I've met many dedicated people. Gary stands out. His perspective is earned the hard way, and APS reflects that depth. For any athlete or anyone seeking clarity, consistency, and a way to perform at their best when it counts, APS provides a powerful path forward. The APS framework is grounded not only in theory but also in a lifetime of real experience across high-performance sport, leadership, and service. APS shows Gary's ability to recognize importance, adapt under pressure, and respond with clarity and purpose, traits he has consistently demonstrated through decades of challenge and change. Built through elite sport, demanding physical work, and real-world leadership, APS offers a practical, earned approach to maintaining performance, resilience, and growth when it matters most.

Peter McConnell
Team USA Surfboat Crew
Holistic High-Performance Coach
Gold Coast, Australia

Gary Wise is exceptionally talented and efficient when it comes to training the mind. His unique approach, built around strength and acceptance, has molded some powerful young minds. Gary's ability to gain your trust and provide creative solutions has helped me beyond measure. Gary has become one of the most reliable mentors in my life.

JC Deacon
University of Florida
Head Men's Golf Coach

Gary Wise is a coach with an expert understanding of elite performance and leadership. He builds a mindset in his athletes that emphasizes "actions matching intent." As a world record holder, Gary has a distinctive ability to convey his experiential knowledge and resilience in a way that few others can.

Roger Capan,
Team USA Olympic Speed Skater
United States Air Force (Retired)

Gary Wise provides uncommon energy and enthusiasm for task accomplishment. He motivates and directs personnel on the complex tasks associated with their duties and responsibilities. His vast experience as a trainer and mentor of athletes is both measurable and highly respected. Although demanding at times to some, his total attention is to instill in an athlete exactly how to attain success.

William R. Rieger, Ph.D.
Colonel, USA (Retired)

Gary Wise is truly remarkable at helping individuals perform at their best. His deep understanding of the athlete's mind, combined with extensive real-world experience, enables him to connect deeply and deliver transformative results. Whether it's sharpening focus, building resilience, or unlocking potential, Gary has an exceptional talent for guiding people toward their peak, both mentally and professionally.

Jack Turner
University of Florida Junior, 2025
SEC Champion 2025
2 x All American
Team USA Palmer Cup Member

When I first started working with Gary Wise, I was immediately impressed by how accurately he recognized my traits and connected with who I am. But Gary didn't just tell me what my specific areas for growth were; he helped me identify them myself, which boosted my motivation to follow the plan Gary outlined. His skill in rephrasing situations and using them for performance learning is incredible. Gary Wise exemplifies excellence in every part of life, and he teaches us how to do the same by aligning us with the best version of ourselves to get the job done!

Joshua Hess
Eastern Michigan University Freshman, 2025
Swiss Golf National Team Member
Notah Begay III Junior Golf National Championship winner 2025

A Dedication of Gratitude

I extend my deepest gratitude to the remarkable individuals who have inspired, supported, and mentored my performance coaching journey over the past 35+ years.

To Geoffrey Scott, your insights and encouragement have challenged me to push beyond my limits, helping me recognize the power of continuous improvement and the impact of thoughtful, intentional coaching. Your everyday resilience and work ethic accompany me daily, even though we have lived in opposite parts of the world for decades.

To Roger Capan, your unwavering belief in my potential and your guidance have been instrumental in nurturing my passion for understanding the factors influencing human performance. Your wisdom and mentorship have consistently inspired me. Everyone who had the pleasure of knowing you will agree that you left this earth way too soon and are missed every day.

To Retired Colonel William Rieger, your wisdom, discipline, integrity, and leadership have profoundly influenced my coaching approach and instilled in me the importance of purpose in everything I strive to achieve. Your dedication to your country and your belief in always "doing the right thing," no matter the circumstances, will forever shape my beliefs and actions.

To my sons, Matt and Chris, the heart and soul of my journey, your support, love, and inspiration have been my greatest motivators. You both continue to inspire me every day, reminding me of the power of passion, purpose, and, most importantly, connection.

Finally, I would like to thank my surf sports friends and lifeguards, most notably Jeff and Mitzi Archer, as well as the YOLO Board ohana, for their unwavering support and countless good times. I also greatly appreciate my coaching team members over the past decade, most notably Grant and Billy, for endless philosophical debates and allowing me to collaborate and coach in a manner that aligns with my values. Above all, I am grateful to the students for their endless challenges, perspectives, and inspiration, most notably the ones who have sought to reach their maximum potential through hard work and meaningful learning. You know who you are!

What began as a journey of physical preparation and focus evolved into a quest for technical proficiency and knowledge, ultimately culminating in today's mind-first approach to training, which will forever motivate me to be the best version of myself possible.

To the first responders, educators, athletes, leaders, and everyday high achievers who recognize that mastery is not defined by talent alone, but by the choices we make in the moments that test us most, this work is for you. With the most profound appreciation, I thank each of you for the knowledge, encouragement, and dedication you have shared with me. Each of you has played a vital role in my pursuit of meaningful learning and my desire to connect with a deeper purpose. Where this journey will end is unknown, but one thing I firmly believe is that by pursuing actions that align with our intent, our connection to the present moment determines our ability to adapt to life's challenges.

With Eternal Gratitude,

Gary Wise

FOREWORD

I've had the privilege of working alongside Gary Wise for the past six years at the International Junior Golf Academy, where we collaborated to build and implement the mental performance training program for our athletes. Over that time, I've seen many coaches, systems, and philosophies come and go. Very few endure. Fewer still actually work. Gary's does, because it's rooted in truth, discipline, and an uncompromising respect for the process.

No Junk Reps is built on a simple but powerful idea: every outcome is the correct outcome for the process applied. That statement alone cuts through much of the noise that exists in modern self-help and athletic development. We live in a world obsessed with results, scoreboards, rankings, and validation, yet frustrated when those outcomes don't materialize. Gary flips the lens. If you don't like your outcomes, you don't need more motivation or talent. You need better systems.

Gary and I share a deep philosophical alignment on mental training. We don't see it as a vague concept or something you "work on when things go wrong." We see it as a structured path, one that requires daily, intentional, high-quality repetitions over time to reach mastery. In this book, Gary clearly and methodically provides that path through a framework the reader will follow step by step: Recognize, Identify, Align, Transfer, and Accept. This structure is the roadmap. It teaches athletes how to become aware of what's actually happening, clarify what matters, align actions with intention, transfer skills into competition, and ultimately accept outcomes as feedback, not judgment, so that growth can continue.

What qualifies Gary to write this book isn't just what he teaches, it's how he lives. He has trained and competed as an athlete his entire life, and that identity hasn't faded with time. Even today, Gary gets up and paddles over five miles every single morning. Not because it's easy. Not because he always feels like it. But because discipline, not emotion, drives progress. Gary doesn't let his emotions dictate his actions; he uses the task at hand to build momentum. That distinction matters, and it shows up on every page of this book.

I've personally watched Gary work with junior golfers and change lives. Not just performance on the course, but how these athletes think, respond to adversity, and take ownership of their development. He doesn't sugarcoat the work. He doesn't sell comfort. Gary tells the truth: this isn't easy, it isn't about feeling good all the time, and it certainly isn't about shortcuts. It's about building a set of processes and systems that you consistently run every day, regardless of how you feel, until mastery is earned.

The moment I truly understood the depth of Gary's impact came during a college signing ceremony at IJGA. As part of the tradition, graduating students give speeches to the junior players and staff. During our most recent ceremony, one of the top junior golfers, speaking to a packed room, looked directly at Gary and said, "I love you, Gary," before breaking down in tears. The room went silent. In that moment, it became clear to me that these ideas couldn't stay confined within the walls of an academy. They needed to be shared with the world.

This book is not for athletes looking for a quick fix. It's for those who have a dream, feel stuck, or sense they are capable of more but don't yet have a clear path forward. No Junk Reps provides that path. If you are willing to follow the structure, apply the tools, and commit to the process Gary has laid out, this book has the potential to change not only how you perform, but how you live and train every day. This book will not only give you the roadmap you need to reach your goals, but it will also inspire you to start the journey and see it through.

Bill Nelson

Mental Performance Coach.

*Olympic, PGA Tour, LPGA Tour, DP World Tour, PGA Korn Ferry Tour, Division 1
Men's and Women's College Golf Teams*

PREFACE

Our world is changing more rapidly and relentlessly than ever before in human history. Technology, information, and artificial intelligence keep transforming how we learn, communicate, and act. As external changes speed up, we must also accelerate our ability to recognize these shifts and adapt accordingly. When we fail to keep up with change, it creates a familiar yet unsettling feeling: the situation has changed, but I did not.

No Junk Reps was written to address that gap.

Whether you're a young athlete striving to perform at a higher level, or a coach, parent, or mentor supporting that journey, the modern performance landscape is louder and more demanding than ever. Distractions are constant. Information is endless. Expectations are amplified. What athletes need isn't more noise, but greater awareness, presence, and readiness. This book offers structure, language, and practical strategies to help individuals quiet their minds, focus their attention, and respond with composure under pressure.

At the core of performance, whether in sport or life, is the ability to manage oneself in real time. A calm, organized mind enhances emotional regulation and creates access to an Optimal Performance State. When unnecessary mental "tabs" are closed, present-moment focus sharpens, decision-making improves, and the athlete reconnects with the task rather than the outcome. Performance becomes less reactive and more intentional.

One principle guides all of my coaching:

"Every outcome is the correct outcome for the process applied."

This is not a passive statement or an excuse for underperformance. It is a conviction that outcomes provide information. They reflect the quality of preparation, decision-making, adaptability, and execution, not personal worth. Before athletes can fully engage with the Adaptive Performance State framework, they must first accept responsibility for the process they bring into each moment. Only then can meaningful growth occur.

As a performance coach working across multiple sports, especially at the elite level of golf, I have learned that technical skill alone is never the limiting factor. Human behavior is. If coaching were as simple as reading thoughts and emotions on a visible screen, the work would be straightforward. Instead, we must interpret the story being told through posture, tempo, movement patterns, and emotional responses. The body never lies; it reveals capacity, resilience, and adaptability.

Every challenge carries a load. Every athlete brings a certain capacity to meet that load. Outcomes are emotionally charged because context matters, but problems arise when we inflate the importance of results that, once in motion, are largely outside our control. In those moments, adaptability decreases, conviction wavers, and agency is lost. The athlete begins to chase outcomes instead of focusing on executing processes.

Understanding how skills are learned, refined, and expressed under pressure is central to solving this problem. The Adaptive Performance State framework organizes performance development into three interconnected settings: Learning, Training, and Performing. Each environment requires a different balance of conscious control and subconscious execution. Skill acquisition is not linear; it is cyclical, contextual, and adaptive. Through deliberate repetition, feedback, and reflection, fragile movements evolve into automatic, resilient behaviors capable of withstanding competitive stress. This framework is grounded in neuroscience and motor learning science, but its application is practical.

The goal is not perfection; it is competence, confidence, and consistency in unpredictable environments. As cognitive load decreases and pattern recognition strengthens, athletes gain the ability to adapt rather than react.

Importantly, the purpose of No Junk Reps is not to reduce the demands placed on athletes. Pressure is inevitable. Resistance is unavoidable. Instead, this work is about expanding internal capacity, developing emotional regulation, strengthening self-awareness, and aligning default responses with the realities of competition and life. When capacity grows, readiness follows. When readiness improves, performance becomes more reliable.

Ultimately, this book is about building the skills required to access your Optimal Performance State more often, not by forcing outcomes, but by refining the processes that create them. Through awareness, presence, adaptation, and conviction, athletes can close the gap between intention and execution and learn to trust the work they have done when it matters most.

Sincerely,

Gary Wise

Professional Golf Association of Australia - Certified Member
International Society of Sport Psychology - Professional Member

Table of Contents

PART 1

A Personal Journey through

the Adaptive Performance State Lens.

*To be successful, you must accept
discomfort, more than want the
outcome.*

CHAPTER 1

How the Journey Began

When I first began writing the concept of Adaptive Performance State (APS), it was never intended to be a personal story, let alone a published book. It started simply as a manuscript, a thesis for a Master's program that was ultimately terminated during the COVID pandemic. My abstract had been approved, and I was ready to formalize what I had long practiced as a coach: a philosophy of human performance grounded in self-awareness, adaptability, and emotional regulation.

APS emerged as a cognitive-behavioral framework designed to enhance decision-making and performance by regulating metacognition and emotions. Rooted in neuroscience, sport psychology, and mindfulness, it addresses the brain's predictive tendencies by promoting cognitive flexibility and disrupting habitual patterns, especially under pressure. The model evolved into five interconnected pillars: Recognize, Identify, Align, Transfer, and Accept, each fostering awareness, emotional labeling, goal alignment, contextual application, and psychological flexibility. These processes enable individuals to transition from automatic reactions to deliberate actions, making APS a valuable tool for self-management. It is effective not only in high-performance settings, such as sports, leadership, and emergency response, but also in guiding those who have no one to turn to through the challenge of managing their perception of a situation. Such situations occur every day: loneliness, exclusion, comparing oneself to others, or, most commonly, the plain anxiety of life created by misinformation, perception, and the unrealistic expectations of life from social media.

Yet now, in my 65th year, I realize that APS was never merely an academic construct; it was a reflection of my own life's unfolding. What began as a theory has become the lens through which I understand my own evolution, both as an athlete and a human being. Fifty years of training and competition across multiple sports have taught me resilience, preparation, and the ability to perform under pressure. But no amount of physical readiness can prepare you for the inevitable moment when your capabilities can no longer meet the expectations of your identity. Acceptance of change must be recognized early. Adaptive cues must be anchored, practiced, and reflected upon daily. And the story we tell ourselves about who we are must stay aligned with the reality of where we are.

Much of the second half of my life has been shaped by the effects of multiple traumatic brain injuries and the persistent challenges of post-concussion syndrome (PCS). These experiences compelled me to confront the limitations of physical willpower and to reevaluate my understanding of performance. Once, I lived in *"zone 5"*, driven, reactive, and fueled by conflict. Today, I exist primarily in *"zone 2"*, measured, mindful, and grateful. Years ago, that would have felt like a concession. Now, it feels like acceptance and wisdom.

Presence, the simple awareness of being here, now, has replaced the old drive to test limits and break barriers as the truest marker of fulfillment. The road to this realization was neither smooth nor free of pain; it was paved with failure, loss, and the hard-earned humility that only time and struggle can bring. Yet within the challenges of injury and recovery, I found a new form of purpose: the space to write.

No Junk Reps, the culmination of years of toil, reflection, and rediscovery, is not a record of achievements but a meditation on lessons learned through failure, persistence, and the pursuit of awareness. The title, born from my long-standing coaching ethos, represents far more than physical precision; it speaks to a life lived with intention. Every repetition, whether in sport or in thought, becomes meaningful when aligned with awareness, purpose, and acceptance.

As the mile markers ahead become fewer, my appreciation for each moment grows stronger. The APS framework continues to evolve, not as a fixed model, but as a living reflection of the ongoing human experience. It is with deep gratitude, both for those who have walked beside me and for those who have challenged me, that I write this chapter of my journey. What began as an academic thesis has evolved into a personal manifesto, a narrative of *recognition, identification, alignment, transfer, and acceptance*. A story, ultimately, of no junk reps.

Your outcome objective is not your absolute best. Our absolute best is not an everyday occurrence; it's a one-time occurrence. However, you can strive to be your best in the present moment.

CHAPTER 2

The 1970s - Recognition

This time period, through reflection, marked the beginning of what I now realize was hallmarked by my discovery of sport. At the time, I had no understanding of what was happening due to my anger and immaturity. However, in hindsight, I see that my life path was unfolding before me without my knowledge or understanding.

Growing up on the Northern Beaches of Sydney, my most distinct recollection is of two particular houses we lived in. One was a hillside house my parents built in Bayview, a suburb just a short distance from Mona Vale's beaches, and the other was a small weatherboard house directly across from Mona Vale Beach. It was in this latter house that my love for surfing and surf sports was born.

In 1972, I discovered golf while living near Mona Vale Golf Club on Sydney's northern beaches. During my daily walk to primary school, I would cut through the property's perimeter. Over time, I started walking along the rough outside the fence and found out-of-bounds golf balls, which I would collect and sell back to the members for about 20 cents each. One day, a local member offered me a job as a caddie for him. To do so, I had to learn how to caddy and get approval from the golf professional. That marked the beginning of my 50+ year relationship with golf. I learned to caddy there, eventually working Saturday mornings caddying for club members. The three most memorable members, even after 50+ years, are Mr. Bruce Padman, a kind man who never spoke ill of anyone; Frank Gardner, a meticulous race car driver; and Paul Murray, a left handed PGA Professional who, to my recollection, also dabbled in real estate. Each of these three gentlemen, in their own unique way, gave me different perspectives on the game and taught me valuable life lessons that I absorbed subconsciously. The highlight of my time at Mona Vale Golf Club was in 1974 when left-handed Professional Paul Murray asked me to be a substitute caddy at the Coca-Cola Classic at the Lakes Golf Club in Sydney. Paul ultimately lost in a playoff to Bob Shearer. Also in that playoff was Ted Ball, whom I had the pleasure of teaching alongside 16 years later, when we both worked with Mr. Geoff Scott, the former two-term President of the Professional Golfers' Association of Australia.

1974 - Suddenly, I found myself moved to a farm outside Alstonville on the far North Coast at age 12, just a few weeks before high school. The anger of being taken from the beach and forced to live on a farm created a deep internal dissonance, as I felt like a hostage to farm life. This was the start of a long, often dark period in my life, during which I frequently displayed the worst in myself for much of the next thirty years. Looking back, I recall having no joy or love in my life. I became increasingly hostile towards my Dad, and my defiance became a behavioral issue at school, at home, and everywhere else.

At 13 or 14, I started being driven by my Mum, hitchhiking, being picked up by surf club elders, or walking 2 miles to catch the bus to Ballina for surf club activities such as patrols and surf carnivals.

1976 - At this point, I developed a strong internal passion for the *"training"* side of sports. It didn't matter whether I was hitting a squash ball up and down the wall, working on depth and precision, swimming laps at the pool focusing on relaxed breathing, ins and outs on the race board or surfski feeling the runners under the craft, punching the heavy bag, running laps on the beach, or playing golf, there was something inherently rewarding about reaching new milestones. This drive led me to improve quickly and also sparked a willingness to push my own limits, which, apparently, on the day of my 15th birthday, resulted in spending that night in the hospital. As I recall, it was the 15-and-under surfski final at Ballina Lighthouse and Lismore Surf Club's annual carnival. I was in the lead pack as we approached the wave area. It was a choppy surf at low tide, about shoulder height. The learned strategy was not to charge the wave and surf down the front but to stall and wait for the wave to break, then paddle in hard on the back of the wave. Apparently, I did not receive the memo, or perhaps I didn't follow the instructions, but seeing an opportunity to win, I charged down the face of a set wave as the other paddlers dug in and let the wave break. The nose of my ski hit the sandbar, then the ski broke, and I ate the front of the ski. The next thing I remember was being taken to the hospital with facial and neck injuries. However, it appears that my bold attempt at winning was a spectacular failure.

During this time, golf re-entered my life as a way to both escape working on the farm and serve as another competitive outlet. After a brief period of just playing freely with other junior golfers and surf club members after school, I realized I could play well, especially since on-course practice was my main option, unlike today's junior golfers. This prompted me to take the train from Lismore to Strathfield in Sydney to compete in the U16 division at the State Championships. Surprisingly, I came away with a win.

At the beginning of Year 11, I transferred from Lismore to Ballina High School, where I started spending more time at the beach and playing sports like rugby, surf events, squash, and golf. Although my anger issues continued, the camaraderie of sports was helpful. Still, while having friends was great, I often felt a strong pull toward solitude, especially when away from the farm. I had played rugby league at my old school, and at the new school, I met a rugby player from the local club whose father was the club president. Ian Arrighi, known as "*Ernie*," introduced a new possibility. While playing in the men's reserve grade rugby as a Year

11 student might have boosted my ego, looking back, it may have also intensified my ongoing anger issues.

Over the next two years, I immersed myself deeper into competitive sports, often for the wrong reasons. My father saw the pursuit of sports as a complete waste of time and in no way was inclined to help or encourage me. This only fueled my obsession. By year 11 of high school, I found myself playing reserve grade rugby on Saturdays and getting the absolute crap beaten out of me playing against fully grown men at a mere 160 lbs., wringing wet. These beatings prompted me to learn boxing, so I could be better equipped to fight back. This cycle of behavior was difficult for my mother to understand, and I later clearly regretted causing her such pain. In August of 1978, we wrapped up the Far North Coast Rugby season by winning the Reserve Grade Premiership, and I was named Ballina's Most Improved Player, an award that finally gave me a sense of pride in receiving.

At this point, my true passion in sports had shifted to surf sports; it didn't matter whether it was shortboard, longboard, body surfing, surf mats, or surf lifesaving races, as they were affectionately called. Some of the rugby old boys who were members of the surf club were *"boaties."* Boaties were a special breed amongst the surf lifesaving club members. I remember Eion Johnson, known as *"Big Jonno,"* who was a rugby player and a boatie. Soon, he and Rugby Coach Lomax, also known as *"Slippers,"* would play key roles in the next chapter of my sporting life. Not only did I love surf sports, but the time spent playing also gave me a sense of belonging. I started staying in the bunkhouse at the surf club for many nights. I could surf until dark, we often had bonfires, and it was a hangout for many local kids. With this environment, trouble also crept in; drinking became common because there wasn't much discipline at the club, as long as you respected the elders. If you rowed surfboats, competed in surf carnivals, or played rugby, they would keep you in line.

Although I didn't share the same passion for rugby as I did for surf sports, I valued the confidence it gave me to stand my ground and fight if necessary. The mentorship from a few of the old boys (the aforementioned *"Slippers"* and *"Big Jonno,"* along with another legendary nickname character named *"Box Head"*) took me under their wing. It taught me life lessons the hard way.

"Till the End." During a trip to the Gold Coast, about three hours north of Ballina, I got the words *'Till the End'* tattooed on my arm. It symbolized, at the time, my readiness to fight for my place, a mindset I thought at the time would be my mantra till the end. Today, however, its meaning has evolved to represent my current purpose: to fight for others and inspire in a way I wish I had been influenced in the late 70s.

In January 1978, I earned a Surf Life Saving Association of Australia Instructor's Certificate. At that time, it felt like I had found a purpose in teaching surf skills to younger kids and maybe even a sense of fulfillment.

My senior year of high school continued to reflect my previous year. By then, my parents had sold the farm and were renovating a house in Ballina, overlooking the water. Unfortunately, my relationship with my father remained unchanged. We struggled to find common ground, and regardless of my sports achievements, I never gained his approval. It just wasn't meant to be. A deeper reason for writing this book is that I always felt I lacked someone to talk to. During those years, admitting you needed help was seen as a weakness, and as a young rugby player, I would never admit to feeling vulnerable. Instead, I did whatever it took to meet the elders' expectations. Today, if just one person benefits from the APS framework by recognizing when a course correction is needed in life, writing this book will have been worthwhile.

Upon finishing high school, I knew my time in Ballina would end as soon as possible. I had saved some money and planned to buy the family

EH Holden Station Wagon and drive back to the Northern Beaches of Sydney, to find the life that had been taken from me six years earlier.

CHAPTER 3

The 1980s - Identify

While the 1970s were characterized by anger and closed-mindedness for young Gary Wise, the 1980s marked a period of self-identity cultivation. Once again, primarily due to my stubbornness and closed-mindedness, I remained unaware of the blessings and gratitude owed to those who had preceded me in life and to those who were soon to present themselves.

I had returned to my roots at the Northern Beaches of Sydney. Now what? With very little money, no job lined up, and no chance to attend university since I had essentially distanced myself from everyone, it was time to buckle down, find a job, and start taking care of myself as a recently turned 19-year-old adult. One great thing about surf clubs in the 70s and 80s was that there was always someone who needed a willing worker for labor jobs on construction sites. For someone who loved training, it became almost a way to get paid to train.

1982 - Years earlier in Ballina, I suffered two major injuries: one to my left knee during a football game, and a more serious injury to my neck from an incident on my 15th birthday. As often happens with injuries that are not properly treated or not treated at all, both would come back to haunt me. During physical therapy at the Australian Sports Medicine Federation clinic at Narrabeen Lakes, I was introduced to the opportunity to study to become a certified Sports Trainer. Unbeknownst to me at the time, this would be the official beginning of my passion for sports performance. Sports Medicine Australia offered early forms of remote learning certifications to young, up-and-coming trainers at the Australian Institute of Sport (AIS) satellite performance and physical therapy/rehabilitation facility, the Sydney Academy of Sport and Recreation. This, in conjunction with the Australian Sports Commission, which was established in 1985, served as the foundation of my ongoing education, a resource for which I have been fortunate enough to have access and support to this day.

1984 - Golf's return to my life happened after high school. During that time, golf faded away as my focus shifted to becoming a certified athletic trainer and personal trainer, earning a living, and competing in other sports. When the surf wasn't good, and I had some free time, Narrabeen Golf Range became the perfect place to hit some balls with my friends. My background as a skilled golfer didn't go unnoticed by Mr. Geoff Scott, who owned Narrabeen Golf Range and Learning Center. While his initial reason for introducing himself to me was not my sound golf fundamentals, it was to ask me to stop hitting drivers into the backyards of the houses behind the range. Soon enough, Mr. Scott became a mentor, and his knowledge and guidance had a profound influence on my golf career.

Opening the door to a new future.

During one of our regular conversations, Geoff Scott mentioned to me whether I would be interested in becoming a trainee Golf Professional. The timing was perfect; I had injured my knee again, which required surgery, and my job as a personal trainer had moved me to their new gym, which was a significantly longer drive than I had become accustomed to. I was intrigued by the opportunity. There was only one problem: you had to be a member of a recognized golf club and have an official handicap of 4 or better. I did not meet either requirement. My play had only been social, and joining the club had not even crossed my mind. At the time, unknown to me, Mr. Scott was the President of the Professional Golf Association of

Australia and was better qualified than anyone to guide me through the nuances of the endeavor I was about to undertake.

Becoming a trainee golf professional in 1984 happened to coincide with the launch of the PGA of Australia's new education program, led by Mr. Max Garske. This program was designed to set the foundation for generations of young PGA of Australia members through a learning framework. The qualifying standard at that time, if my memory serves me correctly, was to break a target score of 300 for 72 holes, in back-to-back 36-hole rounds. The venue was Concord Golf Club in suburban Sydney, and little did I realize what a black sheep I was, lol… For the previous six or seven years, my competitive golf mainly consisted of a few club competitions to establish my handicap and Pennants matches (match-play competitions between clubs within your region). Even my participation in these was as a substitute, as I had only joined Mona Vale Golf within the last six months. Somehow, I managed to navigate (a more appropriate word than swashbuckle) my way around the 72 holes and secure a score that qualified me for the interview process to become a PGA of Australia Trainee Golf Professional.

Throughout my formative years, the traits that might have been attributed to young Gary Wise were perceived as undisciplined, angry, and stubborn. In reflection, these traits were deserved. My first step toward change was undoubtedly influenced by Geoff Scott *"Scotty"*, who recognized that, beneath my rough exterior, there might be qualities that could be developed positively. But how? I soon learned that this was achieved by giving me responsibility and a sense of purpose. His willingness to take a risk on me and guide me into professional golf, despite my limited track record, stemmed from his visionary outlook. The next few years as a PGA of Australia trainee would unfold as the greatest opportunity to learn the craft of golf from my boss at Long Reef Golf Club,

John Kelly *"JK"*, and from Geoff Scott, who had arranged my traineeship with JK at Long Reef.

JK was in his 60s when he took me on as a trainee, even though I was 24. At that age, starting a traineeship was considered quite old. However, my five years as a certified personal trainer and lifelong involvement in multiple sports provided me with diverse perspectives on learning, training, and practice, which proved very valuable at that moment. At Long Reef, we did not have a driving range or even a short-game practice area, but we did have the greatest learning facility ever, an oceanside links course with every opportunity to learn every golf shot you could imagine. JK was not a man to mince words. When it came to developing my game, the directive was always based around what the golf ball did, not what the swing did. If I could sum up JK's teaching philosophy, he instilled in me it would be: ***"Your hands control your tools, be a craftsman."*** Today, there are not many golf instructors who hold this as their overarching belief. But for me, at the time, it was perfect. It taught me creativity, as Long Reef had become like a giant canvas for exploration.

During the early to mid-1980s, I was very fortunate to become friends with a unique group of highly talented individuals who would become both training partners and lifelong friends. Craig, I'd met at Avalon Surf Club, who went on to become a highly decorated police officer; Mark, an incredibly accomplished sailor; Warren and Craig, who were Navy specialists; and Justin, who was a powerlifter at the time and later became a world-class boxer and trainer, trained together in the gym, usually in groups of 2 to 4. Our training ethos was pretty much ***"train hard or go home."*** It was a no-nonsense approach, and some of the feats Justin and Mark achieved back then motivated me for decades. For me, it was the ultimate lesson: my attempt to become a golf professional while still playing squash, rugby, and rowing surfboats was entirely counterproductive to mastery. Each of my mates was highly focused and skilled within their own domain, while I was still caught in my habitually narrow-minded mindset of trying to prove I could do it all. It became clear that I needed to focus on just two sports: golf, which would require the most time and effort to master, and surf sports, which I would always need to be part of my life because of my connection and sense of belonging to the ocean, an experience that has stayed with me for life.

1988 - Discovering Long Driving is a thing. Within the ranks of golf, there is a subset of unique characters that, over the next 10 years or so, I would meet and travel the world competing with and giving exhibitions. The world of long driving was truly a home to some of the most interesting and diverse groups of individuals. Most were not professional golfers, but they all had a gift for hitting the living crap out of a golf ball. At the time, the best of the best competed on two different stages, both based in the United States. The Michelin National Long Drive Championships and a soon-to-be-formed organization called the World Power Golf Association. Discovering long driving also coincided with my joining Geoff Scott's team of PGA instructors at Narrabeen Golf Range and Learning Center. Not many places in Australia at the time could have provided the sheer volume of golf balls hit or the instruction offered at Narrabeen.

In so many ways, Scotty was a visionary in Australian golf. He was the current President of the PGA of Australia and had a wealth of knowledge and experience on the game and its opportunities. I had won several long drive events in Australia by now. I had just won the PGA of Australia long drive title at Sanctuary Cove in Queensland when I received a fax from the aforementioned World Power Golf Long Drive Association, inviting me to the United States to compete in a planned event offering $100,000 for first place, as well as if memory serves me correctly a future long drive eight event tour across the southeast of the United States. This seemed like an unbelievable concept, you mean to pound a little white ball as far as possible, and we could win money of this magnitude? Hold my beer…

While golf was now truly embedded as my job, it was about to turn into a career, though not through the usual routes. I was still an outsider among golf professionals. I continued playing rugby whenever I could, though now less often because my busy schedule made structured training impossible. I also continued to row surfboats at the highest level with the Bungan Beach Surf Lifesaving Club. Over the years, under Ross Jorgenson *"Jorgo"*, Bungan had become one of the strongest surfboat crews in the country, just as he had done with the Warriwood crews before Bungan. Jorgo was ahead of his time in coaching; his use of drills to develop technical skills was probably unmatched in the early to mid-1980s. However, it was an introduction Jorgo was about to make to me that would change the direction of my life forever. It was the first week of April 1988 when our Bungan surfboat crew finished a very disappointing third at the Aussies, the national surf lifesaving championships. Jorgo invited me to play golf at his club with a guest from the United States. The guest was West Kinander Jnr, an executive at his family's electrical manufacturing company based in Chicago. He was also a board member at Medinah Country Club, located just outside Chicago, and a member of the prestigious Western Golf Association.

Medinah, within the United States golf hierarchy, ranked among the very top venues. Medinah had three distinct 18-hole courses, including the famous Course 3, which was set to host the US Senior Open later in 1988 and the US Men's Open in 1990. Unbeknownst to West, I was a golf professional; all he knew was that I rowed surfboats on Jorgo's crew. Likewise, I knew little about his pedigree. We only knew we were both playing golf at Monash Country Club, a beautiful course on Sydney's northern beaches, with a fourth member who was an acquaintance of West and Jorgo. Of course, Jorgo had framed the setup a little differently for both West and me. After 18 holes of good banter, West asked me one question: ***"Do you have a passport?"***

Four weeks after my fortuitous meeting with West Kinander, I was being picked up at Chicago's O'Hare International airport by Mr Kinander's driver and being taken to his beautiful family home in the estate directly opposite the famed gates to Medinah Country Club. He was to allow me the privilege of staying in his pool house and to provide me with an Anniversary Edition 1978 Chevrolet Corvette L82 to drive to and from a playing/teaching position he had secured for me at the exclusive Green Acres Country Club in Northbrook, Illinois. Full access to Medinah Country Club, a beautiful pool house to live in, and a Corvette to drive to a great job. But the one *"perk"* that may have had the most influence on my life was the opportunity, through a member of Green Acres, to train at a gym called The Deerfield Multiplex, a facility that served as the practice center for the Chicago Bulls.

As an athlete with no prior basketball experience beyond casually watching the game and being a low-skilled participant in pick-up games, I found it truly amazing to observe the fascinating dynamics between players' individuality and coaches' unique traits. At the time, while many were predicting their future success, it was only clear to me that they were incredibly talented individuals. As time passed and Phil Jackson established cohesion, they evolved into a team for the ages. It all seemed surreal that this would be my summer home and a place I would visit many times in the years to follow until West's untimely passing.

Our perception of the situation often dictates our response (action), not the situation itself. Choose an action that you will be proud of tomorrow.

CHAPTER 4

The 1990s - Alignment

The years after I first arrived in the United States truly felt like an adventure. The World Power Golf Association (WPGA) Tour had just launched, and the U.S. golf scene offered something for everyone. You could play mini-tour events in Florida and stay in one place, travel to compete in State Opens, play college golf, or test your skills at qualifiers for the newly formed Ben Hogan Tour, or even Monday qualifiers for the PGA Tour. Golf in America seemed to present endless opportunities. I chose to settle in Florida in April 1991; it was the base for the World Power Golf Tour, and at the time, I was able to secure sponsorship to travel across America and around the world, earning money just to hit a little white ball as far as I could. How was this possible? The athletes competing on the WPGT also had plenty of opportunities to play, tournament play, scrambles, exhibitions, and even a nearest-the-pin contest on the 18th hole at the Don Shula Resort in Miami. That hole is a 426-yard par 4, if memory serves me correctly, and was won by Mike Gorton with a shot about 20 feet away. Mike, a five-time world long-drive champion, who couldn't get out on the course to play a money game often enough, remains a good friend today.

Like all good things, these times eventually came to an end. The World Power Golf Tour gave way to their greater interest in golf club component development, and thus a new chapter began. The timing was again fortunate for me, as all the travel over previous years meant I was away from my first and forever love, surf sports. Every Australian summer, I was lucky enough to go home and continue rowing surfboats, surfing, and living on Sydney's northern beaches. Thanks to Geoff Scott, who always made a spot available on his team, I was able to return to Narrabeen and spend the summer at home. However, this annual trip back and forth would soon come to an end, as the decision was made to settle in Florida and pursue my golf career in earnest.

For me, alignment came in the way of recognizing the importance of structuring a life in the US where I could both pursue my career and live the beach life that I had always loved. Over the previous years, *"chasing the carrot"* had become hypnotic to me. I had lost sight of my true identity, and being aligned with those things that had previously brought me solace had been forsaken for more egotistical pursuits. It was time for the first recollectable reset in my life. I had become accustomed to running home every year to my safe place. Now it was time to build a life in the US that incorporated all the components that were important to me. I set up camp in Destin, a quiet fishing village in the Florida panhandle. It was a chill place you could detach from the rigors of life on the road and paddle, occasionally surf, and the World Power Golf Association had set up a golf school at a new nine-hole, fully lit, beachside course and range.

With the World Power Golf Association turning its attention to golf club component development and instruction, more doors opened. Having spent most of my life as a highly competitive athlete in more than half a dozen sports, and as a personal trainer and golf instructor, my lifetime true passion was becoming increasingly clear: I was fascinated by human performance. With the WPGA now turning its focus to golf club component development it was a new opportunity for me to pick up a fascination that many years prior, John Kelly had instilled in me in the workshop of Long Reef Golf Club where he would have me annually replace the binding *"whipping"* of all the members woods along with recutting the score lines and lacquering them.

Next thing you know, we were building custom sets using frequency-matched shafts and storing heads in bins weighed to the gram in a sleepy little Florida panhandle village named Santa Rosa Beach, under the name Javelin Blue. Named after the distinctive radiant blue shafts that we were building our clubs with. At the time, it reminded me of coastal New South Wales, Australian towns we would spend the 80s travelling to for surf trips. Except for one thing, the surf in the Florida panhandle was small, rare, and inconsistent at best. As it always appeared to be when it came to golf in Florida and the US, the opportunities were everywhere. This concept of equipment frequency matching was very new and ahead of its time. It was labor-intensive, impractical or even inefficient at a low-volume output level compared to mass production. Still, it would prove to be only a niche market not easily overcome in gaining acceptance among the larger OEM manufacturers. While all recognized the benefit of a custom-built set, especially for better players, the economies of scale were unfavorable. In the years to follow, most manufacturers would go on to develop custom club kits so they could demonstrate to customers the variety of clubs to suit their diverse golf population, but lie angles, limited shaft flexes, and weighting options, along with head design variety, would become more the norm.

1994 - By now, I had grown somewhat accustomed to life on the Emerald Coast, which is what our region was called. In February that year, Shanah, my son's mother, and I got married. We had met in Destin a few years earlier, and now we were about to build our first house there, one block from the beach. This marked the beginning of raising our two sons, first together and then apart. Looking back now, of course, there are many things you wish you could have done better in life; being more patient, aware, and accepting during this time would have been at the top of my list. No matter how much you prepare for something, experience remains our best teacher. If writing these memoirs and this book helps just one person become a better, more aware version of themselves, it will be worth the effort. Years later, we can look back, now as grandparents, and see how fortunate we are that our sons love us both and how strong and kind they have become.

1995 - Our first son is born twenty-four hours after Hurricane Opal slams into the Florida panhandle. Shanah and I received the unexpected news from the hospital in Fort Walton Beach that we had to take our newborn Matthew and leave. Why? Because the hospital was going to be used as an evacuation center for displaced locals as Hurricane Opal approached. While it seemed impossible to fathom, we had to think fast and logically. Yes, we had a solidly constructed new house that would probably withstand the rigors of a Category 3 hurricane, but was it worth the likelihood of days, if not weeks, without power or probable flooding? It was not, so we decided to drive her and newborn Matt to her parents' house in Mississippi. Typically, about a 4-hour drive, on this day, in driving rain and tropical storm conditions, with thousands of evacuees, who knows. So many other considerations, was there going to be petrol available? Would there be phone service or power along the way? There was only one way to find out. We were prepared as much as possible, and with only a few challenges along the way, I was able to drop them off safely and turn around and head back to the house where we had been forced to leave Spudly, our beloved Staffordshire terrier, locked in the house. It would be 10 days before I saw them again. For me, 10 days of removing hurricane debris, without water or power, but when all was said and done, they were able to return home, and we turned our attention to our new life, raising our son.

For those living along the Gulf of Mexico in Florida, surfing in winter was occasional at best, and summer surf was mostly flat except during tropical storms. Tropical storms and hurricanes would inspire many of Florida's most dedicated surfers to chase the waves wherever the forecast predicted good conditions. Social media hadn't been invented yet, so we depended on newspapers and TV weather reports for wave updates. Around that time, a good mate of mine from Australia, Peter Hickey, came up with the novel idea of bringing the winning surfboat crew from a nationally sponsored Surfboat Championships in Queensland to the United States to promote the sport and attract more competition back home. While surfboat rowing was part of the surf lifesaving culture in many countries, Americans mainly preferred single and pair-dory rowing as the main surf rowing styles. It was never about changing the culture, just about offering more participation options. With this in mind, I started establishing the United States Surf Rowers Association, with the initial goal of forming a crew or crews capable of hosting an annual Aussie surfboat championship and becoming competitive enough to compete in the International Lifesaving Society World Championships.

1996 - There is no greater impact on your life than raising your first child. No words, no courses, and not even watching others do it can fully prepare you for the changes you'll experience. The internal shifts that a simple smile or gesture can evoke are beyond words. It truly is a special time. For me, many of these feelings were so distant from my previous state of being. Becoming a dad had the most profound effect on me. Even though becoming a dad was by far the most important thing to me at the time, the itch to get back on the water grew into a necessity to act. Fortunately, I was given the opportunity in the summer of 1996 to jump back into a surfboat after a few years away. Peter Hickey was planning to send a strong Queensland crew to California to race against Team America, and we needed to develop a plan to provide some competition.

The boats had already been shipped by container from Australia, the sponsors had handled the logistics, and an event called Pacific Pride was being promoted. Steve DeBever and Pat Kelly, two excellent rowers from California, had previously rowed surfboats with local West Coast lifeguards and were eager to elevate surfboat rowing in the US, so we officially formed and registered the United States Surf Rowers Association, along with Pete McConnell, an Aussie mate from home whom I had known during my Long Reef Golf Club days. Pete was living and working in California, and with Peter Hickey, sweeping us, we began a unique journey that would take us to the World Titles. When we were short a man, we could always find a willing *'boatie'* to jump in and have a row.

We trained together in California when logistics allowed, at Mother's Beach, a convenient location that allowed for technical water in the flats before heading into the open water. For the next four years, we prepared on our own and met occasionally before a big race to spend time together finding our rhythm as a crew. Compared to how regular crews train around the world, it seemed unlikely to work; however, for us, it was simply a necessity that was surprisingly effective. Over the ensuing years, we managed to have some great races with the visiting Australian crews. The three-race series would always end 2-1 in favor of either nation, including trips to Australia to compete.

In 2002, we competed in the International World Lifesaving Championships in Daytona Beach, Florida. More surfboats had been shipped from Australia to the US for this event, and for us, it was going to be the culmination of six years of rowing together in the most unlikely of circumstances. Winning the Master's division was not only a highlight but also spurred us on to commit to two more years together, to venture to Italy in 2004 to defend, and thus began our last chapter of the journey that would see us compete together for nearly a decade. Even though we only came away with the silver in Italy, the journey was a testament to our resilience and love for rowing, keeping this dream alive for so long.

1997 - We are now a family of four, having welcomed our beautiful baby boy, Chris, into the world. What should have been a wonderful time revealed many unresolved challenges. My work frequently kept me away; last year alone, I took eight international and even more domestic trips. I was unaware of the stress this caused Shanah, especially with two children now. My travel schedule needed to change. This realization comes with hindsight, but at the time, I believed that providing for my family was my top priority. Many others around the world likely feel similar strains, often traveling through life with blinders on and misguided priorities influencing their choices. Perhaps, if I had written this book earlier, I would have been more aware and made better decisions. But, as usual, hindsight often comes too late for corrective action.

By now, it had become apparent that custom-made golf clubs were a niche market and that small boutique brands, such as Javelin Blue, would always struggle against the marketing power of industry leaders.

In golf, brand loyalty is a strong form of confirmation bias. It didn't matter to the majority of golfers whether a product was better suited to their game; they would toil away with their preferred brand without considering better options.

For me, however, having had the opportunity to work in and around the PGA Tour, interacting with players, instructors, fitness trainers in the newly developed PGA Tour Fitness trailers, and Tour reps. Through these associations and by observing how the players prepare, I was able to form beliefs about the strengths and weaknesses of the methodologies Tour players use as athletes, compared to those in other sports I'd been involved with, both in training myself and others.

The introduction of the PGA Tour fitness trailers, along with the rise of a rising star named Tiger Woods, forever changed the landscape of golf performance. While the debate over the greatest golfer of all time will always remain unresolved among golf aficionados, one thing is sure. In recent years, a generational shift has been underway, with Tour players placing more emphasis on athletic and functional training than ever before.

This cultural change also led to the emergence of a new performance discipline, with the role of sport psychologists in preparing elite golf athletes. For me, these shifts were profound and shaped my future. I began viewing athlete preparation from a more holistic perspective, leading to the development of the Human Maximum Performance training protocol. Specializing in elite golf athlete development with an integrated approach to mental, physical, and strategic performance. Along with coaching services that extended into the realms of open water athletes in rowing, paddle sports, and surf lifesaving. I found true alignment.

The next phase was both brief and demanding. I was recruited to join the Ben Hogan Golf Club brand under Spalding's new ownership. Jeff Sheets was appointed Director of Golf Club Development and brought me on as the R&D and Custom Club Manager. My position was based at Spalding's equipment test facility in Palm Beach, Florida, where I oversaw component testing and performance analysis using robotic and human testing protocols.

Additionally, I facilitated PGA Professional certification in custom fitting through the PGA of America and managed club fitting for Ben Hogan staff and advisory players. This was an exciting period in my career trajectory, but also because I could travel less and be based in our beautiful new home in Palm Beach Gardens. We proudly owned a stunning four-bedroom house on just over an acre in the gated Steeplechase community. What could go wrong?

At first, everything seemed to be going well at work and at home. The boys were 3 and 1 years old, and Shanah didn't need to work. However, the elite Ben Hogan brand, now owned by the more *"big box"* oriented company Spalding, was misaligned. No matter how brilliant the concepts or beautiful the clubs the Ben Hogan brand produced, the stigma of the Spalding name always seemed to cast a shadow over the once esteemed Hogan name.

This was especially clear during the development and release of the Hogan Apex Plus irons. Beautifully designed by Jeff Sheets, tested, and refined by our team, they ultimately didn't receive the response we hoped for. The Hogan name under the Spalding umbrella was beginning to stall. Mr. Hogan had built his brand's reputation on the premise that a club bearing his name was like a fine piece of jewelry and must be presented and cared for as such.

His reputation prior to his passing in 1997 was one of zero tolerance for any quality flaws. As with many boutique golf companies in the past, the Hogan name could not be transferred to higher volume sales. With the Hogan name now associated with being acquired by Callaway Golf, based in California, Hogan began consolidating assets, and our test facility in Palm Beach was one of the first to be sold. Faced with the choice of relocating to Chicopee Falls, Massachusetts, pending the sale to Callaway, or returning to Destin, Florida, where we had just left over two years earlier, we chose the latter, and thus a new chapter began.

Acceptance allows one to recognize an outcome for what it is, regardless of the result, a moment, successful or otherwise.

CHAPTER 5

The 2000s - Transference

Over the past decades, my life has been centered around identifying as an athlete and the relentless skill acquisition towards mastering my craft as a Performance Coach. Now was the time to transfer this learning and these skills to supporting my young family back on the Emerald Coast of Florida. While it was going to be challenging to start my coaching practice from scratch in a relatively small community, I was confident that the knowledge gained over the previous years would lead to success.

2000 - As previously mentioned, our Team USA surfboat crew experienced some success against the Aussies, and we were now dedicated to competing in the upcoming World Championships in Daytona Beach. I faced a dilemma: my left knee had been operated on multiple times without success, and I was approaching the need for replacement surgery.

By early 2000, my Concept2 times, used as the standard in rowing testing, were quite respectable for 500, 1000, and 2000 meters. However, to fulfill my commitment to the team and prepare for the World Championships, I decided to schedule the surgery. My goal was straightforward: recover with new knee components, return to training, and try to regain and surpass my previous times, despite the uncertainty of how my body would adapt to the new parts. Fortunately, the healing process went smoothly, and I was able to resume training, ultimately setting two world records in the Master's division for 500 and 1000 meters.

Along with these records, and as previously mentioned, our competing in the 2002 and 2004 World Championships, it was apparent that my time devoted to surfboat rowing was coming to a regrettable end.

2003 - Black Sunday is a lasting memory along the Florida Panhandle, a tragic event impacting many lives, from the beautiful white-sand beaches of the Emerald Coast to families who lost loved ones and locals who didn't return home.

For my oldest son, Matt, and me, the day after Black Sunday marked a key moment in trust and skill transfer. Both Matt and his brother Chris loved the beach: skimboarding, surfing, paddling, or body surfing, it didn't matter; they loved the water. On that particular afternoon, Matt, then 7, was riding the waves from the previous day's tragedy. The surf at Pomapo Joes was about 3 feet, and he enjoyed it on his 5'6" soft rail surfboard. Both boys were skilled swimmers, practicing regularly in the pool and doing lifeguard drills like underwater rock retrievals.

Just before 6:00 pm, I heard a scream from about 40 yards east of us. Two young people, a boy and a girl, were caught in a rip current, losing their footing as the current pulled them into the gulf. I wasn't surfing but was treading water and pushing Matt into the takeoff zone to catch waves, then body surfing in to assist him in punching back through the waves.

When I heard the scream, I moved to push Matt into the next right-hander approaching them. I told him to aim his board into the wave and have the victims drape their arms across it and hold on. To avoid his leg rope, he was to slip off the back, and either hold the board's back or tread water until I arrived. The sequence went smoothly, and about 45 seconds later, I swam across the sandbar into the rip channel, and we all headed calmly to the next sandbar to stand. We returned the victims to shore, and once the original victims were calm, they walked away with a life lesson.

Twenty-five months later, while surfing Hurricane Rita's leftover waves with Chris, I saw him paddle over to rescue a panicked boogie boarder who had lost her board. These moments made me incredibly proud, not just of the outcome but of how composed both boys remained under challenging conditions, responding systematically based on their training. By age 16, they were working as professional lifeguards at Destin Beach Safety, having spent years as junior lifeguards and eventually representing Team USA at the International World Lifesaving Society World Championships.

2005 - While personally I had overcome having had my knee replaced at the young age of 40 and had sporting success, again my lack of awareness had taken its toll on Shanah and my marriage. Simply put, we were at an impasse. I still couldn't grasp the concept of accepting that there are always two sides to every story, and my relentless pursuit of building a successful coaching practice and winning races had left her more alone than ever.

In early 2005, we separated and divorced. Writing this down for the first time, all these years later and with much water under the bridge, I realize it is almost entirely my fault. Sometimes we are blinded by ambition and drive, and literally have no ability to recognize the importance of things we are not paying attention to.

The next ten years of my life are well documented in the Third Revision of The Concept of Adaptive Performance State. I would shift my focus from the four things I loved so much for many years, family, golf, surf sports, and performance coaching, to being a single dad, and building a Beach Safety/Surf Rescue program from scratch along the 26 miles of what had been nationally recognized as America's most dangerous beaches on the Emerald Coast of Florida. This was to prove the most challenging time of my life. I would have to draw on all the lessons learned over the previous years, the relentless pursuit of overcoming obstacles, strategic planning and design, coaching on physical and mental preparedness, and, most importantly, leadership. All while learning the ways of being a present dad after our recent divorce. This was the time when the entirety of the concept of Adaptive Performance State would be transferred from a theoretical construct to action, first and foremost being the best Dad possible and building a professional life-saving organization.

2006 - With our surfboat rowing days recently behind us, I felt the desire to try something new. Standup paddleboarding (SUP) seemed to be the perfect craft for the Beaches of South Walton. Once again, luck played a role as a new stand-up paddleboard company emerged within two miles of my house in the unlikely area of Santa Rosa Beach, Florida. Jeff Archer, whom I now proudly call one of my closest friends, had just started **YoloBoard**. The timing couldn't have been better for me. Whether there was surf or not, it didn't matter. You could paddle surf, do a long-distance training paddle, head out into the bumps and surf them back to the start, or explore the beautiful intercoastal waterways. It offered the perfect options for surfing, training, and racing. I became hooked quickly.

In 2006, the first race on the East Coast of the U.S. to include a standup paddleboard division took place, and over the next few years, SUP divisions in established races and new SUP races began to grow rapidly. By 2010, there may have been 40 races in the Southeast U.S., with some of the bigger races offering prize money in their elite paddler divisions. Not only did Jeff and YoloBoard provide a competitive outlet for paddlers, but they also fostered a paddling ohana that united people from diverse backgrounds through a shared love of water and paddling. Our Wednesday afternoon and weekend *"Mileage Builder"* gatherings became a special and inclusive event that many participants eagerly anticipate each week. The influx of new paddlers led to greater variety, with many now wanting to go faster, switching to surf skis and outrigger canoes, the long-standing race craft became a popular transition. While prone paddling remained a constant, and was mainly a choice for lifeguards, whose 10′ 6″ boards had been raced in surf lifesaving competitions for decades.

Both my boys loved surfing more than any other pastime or sport, so much of our free time was spent at the beach. They enjoyed learning the skills of every craft and loved being on the water, which was something we could always do together. As our emerging lifeguard agency grew, so did the number of lifeguards getting into paddling.

In its early days, most of our guards had little to no background in surf sports or lifeguard competition; many hadn't even been competitive swimmers. However, in a short time, half of our lifeguard team was paddling and learning new skills that would make them better watermen and women. With every tower and ATV equipped with a rescue board, there was never a reason not to sharpen your skills, and they loved it. I genuinely believe this shared love for paddling fostered an immediate culture among our guards, creating a stronger connection than if it had just been seen as a summer job; they felt like they belonged to something more.

Our brain makes predictions based on past experiences. Every rep performed, successful or otherwise, serves as a reference marker for future growth.

CHAPTER 6

2015 - Acceptance

"Every outcome is the correct outcome for the process applied," Gary Wise.

The years of battling bureaucracy, combined with the fact that both boys had now graduated from high school and were moving on to the next chapters of their lives, had made it apparent that it was time for me to return to my coaching roots. This chapter had run its course. While the years of serving as Beach Safety Division Chief had been fulfilling in terms of all that we had accomplished, the lives we had saved, and the growth that many of our guards had personally achieved, there was an ever-present void. The county had grown exponentially, yet, due to circumstances beyond my control, I was unable to hire more full-time officers, and I must accept this. It had become very clear to me that the organization needed a change, and it was time for me to bid farewell.

I knew I wanted to return to performance coaching, focusing again on a holistic approach to athletic development. This time, however, I aimed to emphasize the mental aspect. My early coaching years were more focused on the physical aspects of performance, followed by a technical phase. Now, I was fully dedicated to what I called a *"mind-first"* approach to learning, training, and performing. This shift was genuinely shaped not only by the experience I had accumulated over the past 40 years as an athlete but also by the valuable lessons I learned from mentors and students. Although the last 10 years as an ocean rescue chief were often frustrating, they also allowed me to coach, train with, and compete alongside many talented and eager young athletes. However, the most meaningful gift was doing all these activities with my sons. Those moments will always be my greatest joy, surpassing any national or world championship, crossing a channel, a surf trip, or a training session.

Due to a series of random events, I found myself in Clermont, Florida, being interviewed for a Director of Performance position at the National Training Center. The phone conversation that prompted me to drive seven hours for the interview was intriguing. It was one of those talks where both sides quickly fell into a natural flow, seemingly with little effort.

However, when I arrived the following week, the person I had spoken with was no longer employed there, and their replacement presented a completely different scenario from what had been previously explained and what I was excited to be part of.

Although the person I spoke to was no longer conducting an official interview, they shared a piece of information that I decided to follow up on. About 20 minutes away was a junior golf academy owned by someone I had encountered before, Gary Gilchrist, and led by Grant Balcke, a golf professional whose name I recognized as a young pro from the PGA of Australia. The lady at the National Training Center offered me a free workout and swim in their lap pool, which I gladly accepted.

So, I set out to visit the Gary Gilchrist Junior Golf Academy at Mission Inn Resort in the tiny village of Howey in the Hills, Florida.

I arrived unannounced in the middle of the students' afternoon training. Not knowing what to expect, I hadn't thought to dress as I had been for the interview prior, but rather very casual. I approached the perimeter of the training ground to observe their activities. Ironically, at that moment, an interview was scheduled for an applicant, but clearly, I was not that person. I was, however, the only one there at the time. Grant approached me, even though I wasn't there for an interview, and we still had an informative chat. His group of students was engaged in golf-specific motion drills guided by the academy's seemingly knowledgeable and confident fitness trainer. Watching Grant's group and three or four other groups of about eight students each train was impressive; it reminded me of athletic development drills at the Australian Institute of Sport, except these athletes were young golfers. I did not speak to Gary Gilchrist, who was busy training an LPGA player alongside the junior groups. I left Grant my card, hoping we could catch up someday, then drove to the beach house I had planned to spend the next few weeks at.

About a fortnight later, I received a call from Grant, inquiring if I'd be interested in returning to sit down with them, as they had a potential coaching opening. Today, at the time of writing this final draft, just over 10 years later, Grant and I are still coaching together in Howey in the Hills. While today the academy operates under a different name, the past 10-plus years have been the most insightful period of learning for me, in the sense of witnessing a greater variety of coaching preferences, learning styles, levels of motivation/discipline, and parenting styles than in the entirety of my previous coaching life.

The importance of listening.

What distinguishes a young athlete's developmental path in determining their trajectory, story, and destination? The answer depends on who you ask. The truth is, confirmation bias causes everyone to form an opinion, whether it's based on facts or not. From a high-level view, it seems straightforward, but in reality, the most talented 12-year-old I've seen didn't end up playing in college. The most talented 12-year-old outside my observation might not even be playing their sport at 16 anymore. There are too many influencing factors.

In this book, I explore the limiting factors that can derail young athletes' potential. If I had to identify one core issue, it would be misinformation.

In today's world of information overload, young athletes face a paradox: they have unprecedented access to knowledge, yet are more vulnerable than ever to misinformation. The constant stream of online opinions, highlight reels, and *"hacks"* creates an illusion of instant mastery, leading to unrealistic expectations for both parents and athletes. Genuine progress, such as changing a swing or refining a technique, requires patience; when results aren't immediate, doubt and impulsive changes often follow. This reactive cycle is fueled by confirmation bias, as parents and advisors seek out voices that confirm their impatience or preconceived ideas of talent. As a result, many confuse talent at a young age as a rite of passage to success, but this is simply not true.

In keeping with this closing chapter's Acceptance theme. The coaching landscape continues to evolve at a rapid pace. With mobile devices and digital influences shaping how we all communicate and process information, coaches must now adapt their strategies more than ever before. At times, we face resistance, whether it's a parent's opinion, an athlete's ingrained habit, or a moment that leaves us scratching our heads. Yet within every challenge lies a choice: how we retrieve information, how we process it through our personal filter, and how we choose to respond. This filtering process has become one of the most valuable tools in my coaching philosophy.

Information can be filtered into three categories:

- Relevant - act on it now, it matters.

- Consider later - relevant, yes, but not necessarily in this moment.

- Not relevant - discard it as noise or "rubbish."

Once filtered, the next step is equally simple. We again have three options for action:

- Change the situation.

- Influence the situation.

- Accept the situation.

These dual processes, filtering and choosing, are foundational to the development of the Adaptive Performance State (APS) construct. APS was created to quiet the noise, to bring awareness back to what truly matters in the moment. It enables one to recognize what is important, identify a course of action aligned with their present moment intention, and transfer that cognition into deliberate, purposeful action.

Ultimately, APS reminds us to accept all outcomes as valid reflections of the process applied. That, in its simplest form, is the essence of the Adaptive Performance State and the theory behind the phrase, **"No Junk Reps."**

In every moment, every repetition, and every decision becomes an opportunity for growth, with no wasted thoughts and no wasted effort. Just learning, adapting, and performing with purpose. For this, I remain grateful to the athletes who trusted the process, to the challenges that demanded adaptation, and to the moments that taught me the power of awareness in action. APS is not merely a concept; it is a reflection of the journey itself, one grounded in acceptance, growth, and the belief that every experience has value.

Throughout my coaching and leadership journey, I've learned that mastery is about adaptability under pressure. The application of the APS framework has evolved to become my core first principle, guiding how I view human potential and the dynamic relationship between one's adaptive ability to transfer intention to readiness and ultimately into a functional, actionable pathway.

APS has demonstrated that excellence depends on coherence, recognizing one's state, regulating emotions, and adjusting strategies in real time, regardless of the realm, whether coaching a golfer or leading an ocean rescue training drill through uncertainty. The key is awareness followed by choice, which shapes performance. APS makes adaptability trainable and resilience a habit.

Performance isn't just about sustained focus but about intentional focus. In golf, it's impractical to stay mentally engaged all the time; top players naturally shift their focus from broad to narrow in a fluid rhythm, adapting to the needs of the moment. Performance involves continuously managing your state, ensuring that your emotional, mental, and physical systems align effectively with your goals. APS acts as a guide, helping you achieve mental clarity and accuracy. Framing influences how athletes perceive cues and interpret situations. Reframing is an active process of adaptation, transforming threats into challenges and mistakes into learning opportunities.

Ultimately, I believe coaching is about exploring and unveiling your inner processes. Recognizing relevance, opportunity, and patterns; identifying specific present-moment intentions; aligning internal and external pathways; and transferring, through adaptive skills, your intention to relevant actions. Once completed, accepting that all outcomes are the correct results for the process applied to learn and move forward. My friend Phill McDonald puts it so well: *"The runs on the board are one thing, but it's the lessons that count."* My hope is that **"No Junk Reps"** will give you the tools to reframe your blocks, recognizing them for what they truly can become: opportunities.

Every outcome is the correct outcome for the process applied

Over the past 20 years, as my memory loss has worsened, I've found it increasingly complex to include others in my life. Recalling past events often causes stress, and often, due to my inability to recollect, I feel embarrassed. I am often reminded of the Cherokee story of two wolves, which teaches that everyone has an internal struggle between two forces: one dark, driven by anger and negative, dissonant thoughts, and one light, guided by love, peace, and acceptance. The lesson is that the wolf you choose to *"feed,"* through your thoughts, actions, and attention, will ultimately define who you are.

Today, what I'm most grateful for is my ability to, through meditative breathwork, reframe the dark wolf into a state of mindful presence by intentionally focusing my awareness on the present moment, and through the lessons I've learned and drawn upon.

In writing this book, it has become clearer than ever that the saying *"every outcome is the correct outcome for the process applied"* that I have repeated to myself and students countless times over the past 20 years, or will continue to do so as I strive to be more open to connection and belonging, something one can only achieve through acceptance and awareness.

Mastery is the sum of mindset, skill set, and infinite repetitions of quality. Mastery cannot be achieved without this trio. Mastery is a journey, a mindset that recognizes the present and connects to the journey rather than whether you won or lost today.

PART 2

Adaptive Performance State (APS)

Compilation 2010 – 2025

*Winning is not a result of your
desire to win. It is, however, a
reflection of your connection to
the necessities of the present.*

FOREWORD

I first met Gary Wise in 1985 on Sydney's northern beaches. I was a nervous Year 12 high schooler, playing nine holes with a local golf professional and my friend's new boyfriend at Long Reef Golf Club on the Northern Beaches of Sydney. I had no idea that this bloke would become one of the most influential people in my life, or that our friendship would carry on for more than forty years.

It's a privilege to introduce Gary's Adaptive Performance State (APS), because APS reflects exactly how he lives: with awareness, honesty, and the courage to adapt. At its core, APS teaches us to meet change head-on, to recognize the significance of a situation, respond with purpose, and steady ourselves under pressure. It's a system built not from theory alone but from experience, struggle, and an unwavering commitment to growth.

Across the years, I've watched Gary evolve through rugby, surfboat rowing, professional golf, demanding training, and even as the Chief of the beach-safety program he led in Florida's Panhandle. This program transformed community safety and saved lives. The physical toll has been real, shaped by old rugby injuries and the relentless work of leading from the front. Yet Gary continues to adapt with acceptance and resilience. He lives his message every day.

In my 25 years in the well-being and high-performance world, I've met many dedicated people. Gary stands apart. His perspective is earned the hard way, and APS reflects that depth. For any athlete or anyone seeking clarity, consistency, and a way to perform at their best when it counts, APS offers a powerful path forward.

With respect,

Peter McConnell

Holistic High-Performance Coach

Gold Coast, Australia

PREFACE

If we think of all the components that make up a challenge as the "**Load**," and the other side of the equation as the set of tools available to respond to that load, called "**Capacity**." The objective of the APS framework isn't to reduce the load but to increase our capacity, using the tools to help us overcome resistance and manage the gap between our intention and the desired outcome.

The following compilation is divided into three sections:

1. The Concept of Adaptive Performance State - Abstract © written 2010

2. The Concept of Adaptive Performance State - Revision © written 2020

3. The Concept of Adaptive Performance State – 3rd Edition © written 2024 – 2025

Connect with the present-moment challenge rather than reacting to perception. Recognize if the threat is based on fact. More often than not, there is a solution. Look for the solution, not your predictive outcome.

THE CONCEPT OF ADAPTIVE PERFORMANCE STATE (APS)

2010

CHAPTER 7

2010

One of the most difficult challenges facing an athlete is adapting to change, and/or applying changes while managing the inconsistent nature of their sport. Inconsistency was predicated by both internal and external   factors. As a self-organizing organism, the athlete must have a performance process from which they can create physiological and psychological harmony. The guiding principles outlined in the Adaptive Performance State (APS) concept can serve as a platform for the athlete to achieve this process, as well as their ultimate goal of skill mastery.

What do you want to change or achieve? In the context of what you are trying to achieve, have you accomplished this goal before? These neutral questions are a critical component of your self-dialog in the preparation phase for overcoming daily challenges. Whether it be setting up your weekly training plan, completing a training task, performing a benchmarking challenge, or even reframing a recurring negative emotion. Your thoughts dictate your actions; self-organizing your thoughts towards instinctively being in the present is always your goal.

Whatever the challenge you face, beliefs influence thoughts. Overcoming negative beliefs and primal fears is often the toughest challenge we face in our daily lives. How does your past influence your future? Beliefs are developed at a young age and, often unbeknownst to us, are influenced by memories that are planted early on in our lives. For example, if you are repeatedly told *"not"* to do something. This may habitualize you to focus on what *"not"* to do rather than focusing on what you **"can"** do. This thought process may influence your present state as we focus our attention on what we are doing *"wrong,"* rather than what we are doing **"well"**, or trying to improve.

Whether it is overcoming a performance plateau or reaching a new performance level, achieving functional adaptation requires overcoming any *"block"* that we have in our mindset, including limited beliefs, cognitive dissonance, or low self-efficacy. A mindful athlete's priority should be the diligent pursuit of self-awareness, purposeful intent, and movement patterns (actions) that adapt to the athlete's stimulus.

What is Adaptive Performance State (APS)?

Adaptive Performance State (APS) is an individual performance state. whereby one's APS components (tabled below) are sequenced and aligned, creating functional adaptation and flow.

Awareness State

P-1	**Observation = Assess** internal and external variables, **Responsibility** versus **Desire**
P-2	**Recognition = Interpret the** influencing factors relative to the assessment

Intention State

P3	**Prioritization = Identify** a plan that aligns with the **Stimulus**
P4	**Self-Organization =** Align **Energy** with **Intention**

Conversion State

P5	**Energy Regulation = Conscious** sequential process, aligning all relevant variables
P6	**Rehearsal = Functional Equivalence** of movement (action), to match intent

Function State

P7	**Trust = Execution** process performed free of memory dysfunction
P8	**Flow = Complete** specific movement pattern sequence (timing/balance)

Reflection State

P9	**Acceptance = Reconcile** response (thoughts and emotions) to complete the loop
P10	**Regulation = Reorganize** thinking and emotions towards "what's next"

While this selection may not resonate 100% with your beliefs, no worries. Mindset is as individual as our fingerprints. It is most important, however, that you identify your performance mindset priorities and pursue them with diligence. This pursuit will have a significant positive influence on the physiological and psychological processes that improve your functional performance.

The athlete's intention, when training or competing, is to *"tick"* as many of these performance pillar boxes throughout their event. When faced with cognitive dissonance, you should be able to reframe the moment at will by applying a personal stimulus trigger. Converting this intention into a matching action while managing emotions and thought processes is the final step in creating a successful performance outcome. When training to improve technique, for example, one should prioritize intention, specifically to reframe suboptimal patterns. Reprogramming these suboptimal patterns with biomechanically functional movement patterns, performed with minimal interference from subconscious thoughts, allows for the development of an Adaptive Performance State (APS).

The athlete must have a standard by which they can gauge the effectiveness of their APS. In my belief system, the process of self-evaluation is known as Rate of Perceived Awareness (RPA). This evaluation is conducted by both the coach and the athlete to foster a deeper understanding and clarity for future goal setting. The overarching belief of the RPA is that one is responsible for one's thoughts and actions. This reflection process creates a platform that aligns an athlete's intentions, stimulus, and attention, enabling them to produce a higher level of function.

The goal in closing every RPA process is to develop further the athlete's self-organizing skills, including, when possible, writing down at least one positive thought or a lesson learned. Lessons learned, whether they result from an unforeseen perspective, a poor performance, or a key thought that led to a win, create the stimulus for future improvement. This reconciliation of thoughts, along with constant evaluation of priorities, is the catalyst for the development of one's self-efficacy.

Simply put, the self-aware athlete with purposeful intention, coupled with positive self-efficacy, is better prepared to self-organize and efficiently translate what they imagine into more functional action.

The Concept of Adaptive Performance State (APS) ©

2020

Presence requires awareness,
capacity, and energy.

CHAPTER 8

2020

Purpose

The concept of Adaptive Performance State (APS) is best described as the workspace between one's intention and the varied, often complex procedures that lead to an action. APS could also be referred to as a structured *"mind management sequence"* that serves as a framework for mindfully converting an intention into a functional action pattern.

The APS framework aims to enhance athletes' ability to solve problems, make decisions, regulate emotions, and maintain commitment in life, training, and competitive environments. Furthermore, these functions should align with their self-identity, beliefs, and purpose. By recognizing this intent, athletes can develop skills and cultivate character traits such as awareness, discipline, resilience, and acceptance; these pillars can be the difference-makers in living a life of purpose and mastery.

An athletic movement pattern, such as the golf swing, is considered a motor skill. Motor skills are learned abilities that involve the coordination of muscles and the nervous system to perform specific movements. The action of an effective golf swing involves complex coordination, timing, balance, and fine motor control, all characteristics of motor skills.

The crucial role of gathering information, planning, mental imagery, and decision-making that precedes the voluntary movement of an athletic motion, such as the golf swing, occurs in the prefrontal cortex. The Prefrontal Cortex is the area of the brain that controls higher-order cognitive functions. When we are *"present"* while formulating the intent preceding an action, it possesses *"situational command."* The Prefrontal Cortex remains in control throughout one's intention phase. Task transfer and/or task sharing are essential for efficient movement from intention to action, via a rehearsal process. This sequence of events is not as simple as flipping a switch. Once the prefrontal cortex evaluates the need for a specific action and develops a plan, it communicates with other areas, such as the premotor cortex and the primary motor cortex, also situated in the frontal lobe.

The application of the APS framework is designed to function as a sequence in which the Prefrontal Cortex, located within the frontal lobe, evaluates a situational challenge, considers the consequences, contextualizes one's current experience relative to past experiences, and formulates a strategic response.

When it comes to initiating the backswing within the golf swing execution process, multiple areas of the brain are involved. This includes the primary motor cortex, responsible for executing movements. The supplementary motor area also plays a significant role in planning and sequencing motor tasks. Before or at the onset of a motor skill, such as the aforementioned backswing in golf, the role of the basal ganglia is significant, as this is where stored repetitions of similar actions performed in the past are located.

The application of a systematic sequence of events (APS) enables the prefrontal cortex (often referred to as the conscious mind) to complete the tasks of strategic planning and mental imagery (including rehearsal) before transferring control to procedural memory (often referred to as the subconscious mind) to apply the motor skills required to perform the actions in the strategic plan.

The process of learning the functional motor skill of the golf swing, culminating in playing the game of golf in a competitive environment, is a systematic journey that requires many years of motor skill training and application. The level and consistency with which an athlete can perform these motor skills in a competitive setting reflect the athlete's functional ability to detach from the impulse to consciously control the execution of the motor skill and instead allow the motor skill to occur subconsciously through the acquisition of a stored memory file.

Hypothetically, if one were to divide stored memories systematically for functional recollection purposes, the ideal system would be:

1. **Green files** = optimal performance leading to optimal outcome
2. **Yellow files** = functional performance leading to an acceptable outcome
3. **Red files** = dysfunctional performance leading to a substandard outcome

In a perfect world, one could create an optimal strategic plan, efficiently retrieve the associated green memory file, and activate the required motor skills, while also storing the same acquired pattern for future use. Unfortunately, this world does not exist.

Procedural memory is essentially a part of the subconscious mind, as it stores information about how to perform actions without conscious awareness. This means that the skills and habits stored in procedural memory are automatically accessed and executed below the level of conscious thought, making it a key component of the subconscious mind's functions.

Understanding how the brain functions at this level helps contextualize the sequence of events that one must focus on at each level of learning and application. The ability of an athlete to perform in the present moment directly reflects their responses to current stimuli.

Both procedural memory and the subconscious mind are considered *"implicit,"* meaning they operate without conscious effort or the need to recall the information. Procedural memory primarily stores motor skills and habits, such as riding a bike, shooting a free throw in basketball, or executing a rowing stroke, all of which are automatically performed without conscious thought, aligning perfectly with the function of the subconscious mind once a certain level of skill acquisition has been achieved. The brain areas associated with procedural memory, like the cerebellum and basal ganglia, are also linked to subconscious processing, further supporting this connection. The majority of processes occurring within the basal ganglia happen at a subconscious level. It is essential, however, to acknowledge that skill acquisition is initially learned and stored consciously through the commands of the prefrontal cortex and hippocampus. These new motor skills must be learned, understood, trained, and memorized through drills, progressing from simple to complex and from slow to faster speeds.

The theoretical foundation of the APS framework is as follows:

1. Recognition

Recognition is a state of awareness that prioritizes what's important now. Initially recognizing the source of the information/perception/biases, and relevance, etc. Secondly, interpreting the influencing factors relative to the strategic plan or the impending decision currently pending.

2. Identify

Identify the variables that may influence the objective and decide on a specific strategic plan that will lead to the preferred outcome. This includes awareness of potential risks, conflict resolution considerations, and opportunistic considerations. For example, am I paying attention to something I can control, or am I paying attention to something external that I have no control over?

3. Alignment

Align one's skillset, focus, composure, and emotions in a functional sequence that matches the strategic plan. Rehearse the plan, focusing on replicating the pattern, providing credible feedback, and building trust. The effective transformation of the prefrontal cortex command to procedural memory activation is dependent on one's ability to perform in a state referred to as a *quiet mind*.

4. Transfer

Focusing one's attention on the conscious motor skill activation cue and then transferring it into the subconscious functional pattern (procedural memory) required for optimal pattern acquisition.)

5. Acceptance

Accept that all outcomes are correct for the process applied. Apply the APS framework for learning, task transfer, self-regulation, and return to situational awareness.

Practical Application:

The application of a new pattern of thinking, movement, or behavior change requires understanding, belief, and discipline for the new pattern to become ingrained. The structure of the APS process helps the athlete develop the discipline, resilience, and equanimity necessary to cultivate the adaptive skills required for thriving in a life of actions aligned with their intentions.

1. Recognition:

Whether it is recognizing the functionality or otherwise of a pattern, such as a state or trait, a mindful reset, or simply one's commitment to a decision, recognition is the first step in awareness/self-regulation within the structure of the APS sequence. Recognition should occur at every stage of the APS process, whenever an individual is striving to achieve growth, change, or acceptance, and an adaptive decision is required.

Recognition also involves being aware of the impending challenges and asking questions that will help solve, rather than hinder, the problem at hand. For example, *"Do I have the resources, skills, and efficacy for this moment?"*, or *"Is my intention aligned with my environment?"* All questions can help recognize the priority of the specific task at hand and guide a course for success.

2. Identify:

The effectiveness of the identification step within the APS sequence is predicated on our ability to interpret the information gathered. This includes the compartmentalization of any threats, perceived or otherwise, and the identification of the clear objective at that moment. That is an objective that fits within the scope of your acquired skills and efficacy in similar circumstances. In short, committing to a decision that instills confidence and trust in oneself.

3. Alignment:

Alignment is the final stage of intention before the task of transferring one's vision into action. Awareness of where one's attention is focused in overcoming the present moment's challenge must be recognized. If the attention is not aligned with one's objective, a trained response must be strategically implemented. Alignment takes many forms, including energy, beliefs, skill efficacy, and emotional regulation. For a seamless conversion from a conscious plan to a subconscious action performed in a state of flow, one's commands must be simple, concise, and best delivered sequentially in a pattern that has been rehearsed previously.

4. Transfer:

Successful conversion of an intention to a functional action pattern is a product of the clarity of the commands provided, along with the athlete's technical proficiency, mental skills, emotional regulation, and available resources. These contextual factors, along with environmental considerations, self-belief, situational efficacy, and cognitive abilities, all impact transferability; each has a varying degree of effect on how well skills are transferred.

5. Acceptance:

"Every outcome is the correct outcome for the process applied." One must accept that all outcomes are correct for the process applied; this is rule number one of acceptance. One cannot close the loop on a process and move forward without acceptance. Regardless of one's feelings towards the outcome, it must first be accepted. With acceptance, one can then respond more appropriately. Upon acceptance, one can apply a problem-solving strategy. This problem-solving strategy is best accomplished from a place of emotional composure and, therefore, a clear-thinking mindset.

Significance:

The APS sequence is designed to be a structured process that enables athletes to adapt fluidly to the mental, emotional, and physical demands of their sport, both in training and competitive environments. Adaptation is crucial to success because it influences discipline, skill prioritization, mental resilience, and overall well-being —all vital components in an athlete's ability to *"put in the work"* required to succeed.

The following are factors that are positively influenced by the successful implementation of the APS framework:

Self-Awareness

Self-awareness is one's ability to recognize, perceive, and understand where and how their thoughts, emotions, and actions influence oneself and others at any given time. Essentially, it is a reflective state in which one evaluates one's intentions and actions in relation to a specific situation.

Self-Regulation

Athletes regularly face anxiety (perceived uncertainty), stress (demands outweigh resources), and/or fearful (impending danger) situations, in competition, training, or under the spotlight of public expectations. The successful application of the APS sequence enables athletes to develop effective self-regulation and coping strategies that include relaxation techniques, mental reframing, and focusing strategies. All are designed to help them manage their emotions, feelings, and thoughts and return to a state of optimal performance.

Building Resilience

Adaptation is central to developing mental toughness and the grit required to *"push through"* difficult circumstances, regardless of whether the athlete faces internal or external obstacles. Athletes who can adapt more easily to setbacks, injuries, and failures typically demonstrate resilience. Adaptation fosters a growth mindset, where athletes view challenges as opportunities for growth rather than insurmountable obstacles.

Critical Thinking

Critical thinking is the objective analysis of facts to form a judgment. Critical thinking is a process that is rarely considered during the development of an athlete from a mindset perspective; however, one benefits from cultivating critical thinking skills whenever problem-solving, decision-making, and planning are required. The subject is complex, and there are many definitions. All of which, however, include the rational, unbiased analysis and evaluation of factual evidence. Critical thinking in sports should be systematic to develop consistency within the process. This consistency will lead to confidence and trust in the process. The systemic nature of the process should include consistency in information gathering, rehearsal process timing, and consistency in breathing.

Enhancing Focus and Concentration

Adaptation allows athletes to refine their concentration skills, enabling them to maintain focus at the required time despite internal or external distractions. Procedural memory refers to the motor skills and cognitive patterns that are learned and memorized through repetition. Activation of these patterns results from consciously applying focus and concentration techniques that align with the adaptive skills required at the moment.

Physical and Psychological Recovery

Athletes need to adapt to the physical fatigue and psychological strain that comes with training and competing. Complete recovery strategies, including healthy sleep habits, proper nutrition, and mindful recovery practices such as reflective meditation, journaling, detachment, and focused imagery, are all vital to preventing burnout and overtraining.

Adapting to Different Environments

Athletes often need to compete in unfamiliar settings, facing new conditions (e.g., weather, altitude, crowds, etc.). Psychological adaptation enables one to adjust one's mindset to a state of equanimity and acceptance of the random nature of life and sports, as well as the various environmental challenges that can be faced.

Motivational Shifts

Motivation can fluctuate based on various factors, such as personal priorities, trauma, external pressures, or injury. Adaptation helps athletes remain disciplined and grounded by developing intrinsic motivation attributes and a mastery orientation. This is achieved through techniques like self-talk and journaling, which help reframe negative thoughts and stay present, resulting in a deeper awareness of what's important now.

Applying Mental Tools Training

Mental skills training, including imagery, goal setting, breathwork, focus techniques, and mindful reflection, enables athletes to more readily navigate and adapt to varying situational challenges in life and competitive sports. These strategies allow athletes to focus on the task at hand, build self-esteem, and manage distractions effectively.

Conclusion:

As previously stated, the Concept of Adaptive Performance State (APS) is defined as the workspace for mindfully managing one's self-regulatory processes and decision-making to best facilitate the steps necessary to achieve an action pattern aligned with one's intention and purpose. Simply, the self-aware athlete with purposeful intention, coupled with positive self-efficacy, is better prepared to self-organize and efficiently translate what they imagine into a more functional action.

One final note: The concept of Adaptive Performance State (APS) was first drafted and published in 2010. This revision was a result of the practical application of the original draft and was revised from feedback obtained from 2951 completed post-tournament reports. While the essence of The Concept of Adaptive Performance State has remained the same, there has been a slight evolution in the language used to achieve a deeper understanding and more practical application among the athletes I have had the privilege of coaching.

THE CONCEPT OF ADAPTIVE PERFORMANCE STATE (APS)-THIRD EDITION

Manuscript Edition

Your authentic self is the person you genuinely are deep inside. It's the person who accepts others' opinions without reacting. Authenticity occurs when your intentions, actions, and behaviors consistently align with your rules, beliefs, and values.

CHAPTER 9

The Foundation

The Adaptive Performance State (APS) concept provides a structured framework for achieving optimal performance by enhancing self-awareness and implementing deliberate mental regulation. Its development was driven by extensive experience in challenging environments, including ocean rescue, top-level sports coaching, and emergency response management.

Throughout these domains, a persistent central challenge was how individuals can make decisive decisions, stay composed under pressure, recover efficiently, and adapt to ever-changing circumstances. The APS framework emerged from a practical need to align the theoretical foundations of performance psychology with the real-world operational challenges. Now in its third edition, the APS framework reflects an evolution based on applied neuroscience, field research, and interdisciplinary insights. It offers a model that can be understood, applied, and adapted by coaches, educators, and performers alike.

The formal introduction of the APS construct outside the realm of athletic development occurred in 2006, during the early part of my tenure as Beach Safety Chief for the Beaches of South Walton, Florida. At that time, I had temporarily shifted my focus away from golf performance coaching. I faced the challenging task of establishing a Beach Safety Division for a Fire District along the 26 miles of scenic coastline in Walton County, Florida. This stretch of coastline had previously had minimal formal lifeguard presence and definitely lacked structure under the oversight of a certified Lifeguard agency, such as what became the directive.

The Catalyst

Beach safety operations are inherently challenging by their very nature. This is especially true considering that at any moment along South Walton's 26 miles of Gulf-front beaches, ten coastal dune lakes could routinely breach into the Gulf, making those areas inaccessible during emergencies. The difficulty was compounded by the tragic incident in 2003. On June 8th, now memorialized as **"Black Sunday,"** eight people drowned due to rip currents along the Emerald Coast. The event drew national attention, particularly because of the death of a well-known news anchor, leading CNN to call the region **"America's most dangerous beaches"** (CNN, 2003). Before this tragedy, beach safety infrastructure was inconsistent, and professional lifeguarding was nearly nonexistent in the area.

The following narrative is an excerpt from a detailed incident report attached to the front of the references (attachment 1) and authored by the on-scene commander, Deputy Chief Hughes. On August 30, 2005, just hours after Hurricane Katrina devastated the Gulf Coast, Gary Wise, a trained responder who was acting as a civilian with no official duty that day, received a call from Deputy Chief Hughes. The call was a specific request for him to respond to an emergency rescue situation where the responding agencies, including Sheriff's Officers and Firefighter Rescue Swimmers, were beginning to lose control of the situation. Upon his arrival, Gary encountered multiple emergency personnel caught in a deadly rip current. The rescuers found themselves unable to reach the drowning victim and then unable to free themselves from the outward pull of the rip current. Without hesitation, Gary swam a landline into the surf zone and rip current, securing the trapped first responders and bringing them safely to shore.

At this time, with Chief Hughes, a strategic plan for retrieving the original victim was formulated. This plan was now deemed a body retrieval, as the victim had been floating face down and showed no signs of life from the helicopter's vantage point. The plan was that with the assistance of a lightweight closed-cell foam rescue tube and a single rescue fin, Gary would swim into the rip current out to sea, secure the victim, and return to shore. Ultimately, Gary executed a physically demanding 40-minute retrieval of a 240-pound drowning victim, with the entire process from arrival to completion lasting over two hours in duration. This response, subsequently described by Deputy Chief Sean Hughes as one of the most challenging rescues he had observed in his 21 years of service, resulted in Gary's words, taking the worst beating of his life as he returned through the impact zone connected to the victim. As a result of numerous violent contacts with the sandbar and being *"rag-dolled"* in the turbulent whitewater, Gary sustained injuries that would contribute to his ongoing battle with chronic pain. Ultimately, this led to his awareness of the flexibility in applying the APS framework to his wellness routines, rather than simply viewing it as a performance-based construct.

Transference from Intent to Action

Following the **"Black Sunday"** drownings and the Hurricane Katrina incident, a comprehensive beach safety assessment was conducted by the United States Lifesaving Association and the Walton County Commissioners. Subsequently, the South Walton Fire District was tasked with implementing sweeping reforms. I was appointed Beach Safety Chief, and together we established a professional lifeguard team, introduced a standardized warning flag system, and launched roving patrols to increase public awareness and safety. The goal was clear: to develop a teachable, scalable model that could be integrated into the Fire District's operational procedures and used for training new lifeguards, many of whom had no previous rescue experience. The core mantra,

"Prepare, Recognize, Respond, and Adapt," became the foundation of our strategic approach, building structure, adaptive skills, and foresight in an ever-changing environment.

The Next Unforeseen Challenge Presented Itself

In 2010, the region's 26 miles of Gulf coastline were severely impacted by the Deepwater Horizon oil spill, the largest marine spill in U.S. history (National Oceanic and Atmospheric Administration [NOAA], 2016). Starting on April 20, 2010, a blowout on the BP-operated rig caused the release of over 3 million barrels of oil over 87 days, causing significant damage to marine ecosystems and coastal communities (U.S. Fish & Wildlife Service, 2011). This challenge once again presented our organization with an unforeseen obstacle that required a strategic plan, with minimal time for preparation. The timing was especially unfortunate, as it occurred during the peak of the Spring Break holiday season. The then-APS foundational mantra, **"Prepare, Recognize, Respond, and Adapt,"** served as a structured framework for an adaptive response, demanding flexibility and foresight in a dynamic, high-risk environment.

After a decade serving as Chief, during which the agency expanded in scope and influence, I returned to my origins in high-performance coaching, focusing now on developing junior golfers. APS continued to evolve as a cornerstone of my methodology.

Learning, Growing, and Adapting

The journey through ocean rescue, environmental crisis response, and high-performance coaching revealed a unifying truth: adaptability is not merely a trait, but a practiced skill set rooted in structured awareness and intentional response. The APS construct, forged in the crucible of real-world adversity, has proven to be a universally applicable framework, one that transforms chaos into clarity through the pillars of preparation, recognition, response, and adaptation. Whether navigating the unpredictability of open water or the pressures of elite sport, the lessons learned affirm that success does not lie in eliminating uncertainty but in building cognitive agility and emotional regulation to meet any challenge. At this moment, I have learned that with a growth mindset and the strategic application of the APS structure, problem-solving becomes a transferable competency, one that transcends environments and empowers decision-making and the enhancement of performance-based skills across all domains.

The original Copywritten APS principles were put into practice between 2000 and 2005, tried and tested in a new realm of Emergency Services from 2006 to 2015, and subsequently refined into the structured format that the APS construct is today: **"Recognize, Identify, Align, Transfer, and Accept."** Although the application context shifted from open-water rescue to sports performance, the core purpose remained unchanged. APS functions as a metacognitive and decision-making model to support strategic action and self-regulation.

Metacognitive Awareness

Metacognition, the awareness and regulation of one's cognitive processes, provides significant adaptive benefits in environments that require resilience, creative thinking, and flexibility (Flavell, 1979; Veenman et al., 2006). It allows individuals to evaluate and modify their thinking strategies in real-time, according to the demands of the situation. In high-pressure or rapidly changing settings, this self-awareness becomes essential for effective performance.

A major benefit of metacognitive skills is their ability to facilitate flexible problem-solving. When initial strategies prove ineffective, metacognitively aware individuals are more likely to efficiently pivot to alternative methods, reducing time loss and enhancing adaptability

(Zimmerman, 2002). Additionally, through deliberate self-monitoring, individuals become better decision-makers, especially under stress.

Metacognition also encourages continuous learning. By reflecting on both successes and failures, individuals gain transferable insights that expand their skill sets and improve future performance (Efklides, 2008). This reflective ability strengthens emotional and cognitive regulation, promoting stability and composure in the face of uncertainty or disruptions. As a self-regulatory mechanism, metacognition helps people to navigate present challenges while preparing for future ones. It supports adaptive behavior through learning, reflection, and strategic foresight. Therefore, it is a foundational pillar of sustained adaptability in both personal growth and professional excellence.

Decision-making, meanwhile, involves the intentional selection of actions from various options to achieve a specific outcome. When guided by logical assessment and self-awareness, decision-making benefits from metacognitive insight, resulting in more effective, intention-driven outcomes (Kahneman, 2011). Whether in saving lives, managing performance anxiety, or staying composed on the golf course, the APS framework offers a systematic approach to remain aligned with one's values, strategies, and objectives. In essence, APS ensures that actions align with intentions, a fundamental criterion for adaptive excellence.

CHAPTER 10

Digging Deeper

The Adaptive Performance State (APS) construct aims to facilitate a deliberate shift toward an optimized mindset, thereby boosting performance in both sports and life situations. Engaging in this shift promotes the formation of novel neural connections, improving the brain's ability to recognize patterns and ultimately enhancing habits and self-regulatory skills (Positive Psychology, 2025). Unlike random occurrences, APS stems from specific cognitive processes and emotional regulation techniques used consistently. Unlike the traditional concept of "flow," APS is a trainable and repeatable state that proves effective across diverse situations (ResearchGate, 2018).

Whether in a sports context, responding to emergencies, making crucial decisions, or managing perceptions, APS helps individuals attain a higher degree of awareness, regulate physiological responses, and execute purposeful actions. Employing a structured approach supports the prefrontal cortex, often associated with conscious thinking, completing tasks related to strategic planning and mental imagery (including rehearsal), before transitioning control to procedural memory, which operates more subconsciously (Nature, 2024). This sequence enables the effective execution of motor skills aligned with the strategic plan. To fully benefit from this approach, individuals must understand the value of organized preparation and apply the most effective mental strategies to enhance their performance.

An athlete's Performance Gap refers to the difference between their training efficiency and actual performance in competitions. Bridging this gap requires a deeper understanding of the cognitive and emotional factors influencing the Optimal Performance State (Mandeha, 2024). While an athlete's physical capacity to perform movements remains consistent, the brain's access to the optimal performance state may vary significantly.

Negative thoughts or emotions can interfere with our ability to perceive important patterns that facilitate optimal performance. Therefore, athletes must learn to recognize disruptive thinking, employ constructive responses, and mentally align with their performance objectives. Our repository of both functional and dysfunctional behavior patterns is stored in procedural memory. This type of memory handles the automatic performance of well-practiced behaviors and is usually activated without conscious awareness. However, to access procedural memory effectively, it requires deliberate effort, often called the **"Performance Routine"** in sports.

In constructing any Performance Routine, athletes should prioritize useful information while minimizing irrelevant or distracting content. The effectiveness of finely tuned movement patterns is most consistently supported by structured habits and routines. The unpredictable nature of sports and life does not naturally lend itself to pattern recall or prioritization. Therefore, athletes must intentionally align their routines with performance goals while embracing the uncertainty inherent in competitive environments. This is where embracing the idea that *"every outcome is the correct outcome for the process applied"* becomes instrumental, enabling an athlete to effectively detach from the current moment's result, reset, and move forward to *"what's next"*.

Conducting a SWOT (Strengths, Weaknesses, Opportunities, and Threats) analysis further improves self-awareness and clarifies the path toward specific objectives, whether refining a technical skill, excelling in competition, establishing new habits, or tracking developmental progress (AM World Group, 2025). Implementing a systematic approach is essential to the Adaptive Performance State (APS), ensuring decision-making processes stay organized and effective (ScienceDirect, 2025).

Each APS keyword: Recognition, Identify, Align, Transfer, and Accept, serves as a purposeful foundational step within a clearly defined structure, enabling more accurate prioritization and increasing the likelihood of achieving intended outcomes.

The recognition phase refers to individuals rapidly recognizing opportunities or challenges by utilizing methods that support pattern spotting, trend analysis, and anomaly detection, thereby reducing the risk of oversight. Once something is recognized, the identification phase focuses on understanding the precise nature of the issue or opportunity. A systematic process at this stage enhances the depth of insight and helps minimize misinformation, resulting in more accurate and effective responses.

During the alignment phase, actions are intentionally chosen to reflect specific goals, available resources, and personal or team values. Systematic decision-making ensures that strategies remain coherent and aligned with broader objectives. The capacity to adapt and implement newly acquired skills in relevant contexts, known as skill transfer, is enhanced by a structured evaluation and application process.

Ultimately, gaining individual acceptance of decisions and outcomes is essential for achieving healthy psychological closure and detachment. A structured approach during this phase addresses fears and anxieties related to uncertain results or past failures. It encourages action in *a "trust mode,"* reducing resistance and enabling smoother execution. The systematic APS construct fosters clarity and consistency in decision-making. It reduces errors, improves adaptability, and results in more effective performance in changing environments. For athletes, structured and concise decision-making is a crucial tool necessary for developing and maintaining a higher level of self-regulatory control and increased performance readiness. It helps them adjust to changing conditions while intentionally refining their strategies.

By following a defined framework, athletes can avoid impulsiveness and make deliberate, goal-oriented choices. This method enables the review of past performances, the identification of patterns, and the necessary tactical adjustments. Additionally, a structured process lightens the cognitive load, freeing up mental capacity for execution rather than deliberation. It also builds self-confidence by providing a consistent framework for decision-making, even under pressure.

Connecting present decisions with long-term goals and preparing for a range of possible outcomes provides athletes with the flexibility and resilience necessary for success in unpredictable competitive and life environments. As we continue to explore the APS framework, we will examine how it supports the development of stronger habits and more effective performance systems, as well as the character traits and states it enhances.

CHAPTER 11

Personal Values

Personal values play a crucial role in cultivating both one's self-identity and self-actualization potential. Serving as the foundation upon which an individual's sense of purpose, decisions, and actions are built. They act as a compass, guiding people toward goals that align with their true selves, helping them fulfill their potential in an authentic and meaningful way. When an individual's actions and decisions reflect their core values, they experience greater fulfillment, clarity of purpose, and a sense of alignment with their authentic self (Deci & Ryan, 2000).

Firstly, personal values provide direction and purpose. They help individuals identify what is truly important, offering a roadmap for setting and pursuing meaningful goals. For instance, someone who values creativity may seek opportunities for self-expression, while someone who values independence may pursue goals that allow for autonomy. By aligning decisions with these values, individuals can achieve goals that resonate deeply, giving their lives a clearer sense of purpose (Seligman, 2011).

Secondly, values play a key role in fostering authenticity and alignment. When a person's actions are aligned with their core values, they experience a stronger sense of congruence and fulfillment. For example, a person who values social justice will feel more self-actualized when they contribute to causes that reflect this belief. This alignment between values and actions is essential for self-actualization, as it enables individuals to become their truest selves (Deci & Ryan, 2000).

In addition, personal values fuel intrinsic motivation, which is the internal drive to pursue goals that resonate deeply with one's values. This intrinsic motivation is particularly important when faced with challenges or setbacks. When a person's goals align with their values, they are more likely to persist, driven by a deeper sense of purpose. For instance, someone motivated by the value of growth will continue learning and pushing boundaries even when progress is slow (Deci & Ryan, 2000).

Living by one's values also promotes greater personal well-being and life satisfaction. Self-actualization is not just about achieving external success but also about finding inner peace and fulfillment. People who live in alignment with their values tend to experience higher levels of happiness. For example, someone who values relationships and community will feel more satisfied when they prioritize meaningful connections over superficial achievements, leading to a more fulfilling life (Seligman, 2018).

Finally, personal values guide individuals through the process of adaptation and growth. As people encounter new experiences and challenges, they must recognize opportunities for self-improvement, accept necessary changes, and transfer lessons learned to new situations. This dynamic process of reflection and growth ensures that values continue to guide individuals authentically as they navigate their journey toward self-actualization (Yao et al., 2024).

CHAPTER 12

Procedural Awareness

A structured operational system is essential for all public safety, law enforcement, and military operations manuals. These manuals serve as learning tools and standards of expectations for new candidates, as well as operational and standards guides for all in-service personnel. Similarly, Standard Operating Procedures (SOPs) can benefit athletes by building routines, enhancing mental performance, and developing adaptive strategies.

One key advantage of SOPs is their ability to create consistency and predictability, providing athletes with reliable routines. This predictability helps reduce anxiety, allowing athletes to focus on their performance rather than the stress of decision-making under pressure. SOPs also establish clear objectives, helping athletes understand the stages of their training and competition preparation, thereby enhancing motivation, focus, and a sense of direction throughout the process (Roe, 2021).

Additionally, following a structured routine decreases cognitive load by simplifying decision-making, allowing athletes to conserve mental energy for critical moments. As a result, they can perform better under stress. Through repeated practice of SOPs, athletes can develop positive habits that strengthen their mental resilience and improve their adaptability in high-pressure situations (Birrer & Morgan, 2010).

The framework of SOPs in a team environment fosters a deeper sense of unity, agency, and team mission. It enables the team to interpret strategies, respond to changing conditions, make necessary adjustments as challenges arise, and, most importantly, fully commit to the chosen plan as one. This sense of agency also promotes engagement and responsibility, ensuring that the strategy is followed and adapted in a way that aligns with the team's mission statement (Bridge Athletic, 2021).

SOPs prepare athletes for unforeseen challenges by incorporating contingency plans for unexpected situations. This adaptability allows athletes to respond effectively to changing circumstances during competitions. Moreover, regular performance reviews and feedback sessions are integral to SOPs, enabling athletes to analyze their performance, identify areas for improvement, and refine their strategies accordingly (Roe, 2021).

Incorporating a military-style SOP can enhance not only the efficiency of training and performance routines but also an athlete's mental fortitude. By instilling consistency and clarity in preparation, SOPs foster adaptability and resilience in high-pressure environments. Within a sports performance framework, this approach aligns procedural awareness with personal agency, empowering athletes to consciously understand and control their performance processes. This heightened self-regulation boosts decision-making and self-belief when performing under pressure (Zarcone, 2023).

CHAPTER 13

Adaptive Performance State (APS) and the Nervous System

In sports, the nervous system plays a crucial role in both skill execution and physiological regulation. The Central Nervous System (CNS) governs voluntary movements and cognitive functions, such as decision-making and motor control. Simultaneously, the Autonomic Nervous System (ANS) regulates involuntary processes, including heart rate, respiration, and stress responses. During competition, the CNS enables athletes to execute skills, while the ANS supports performance by balancing stress and recovery mechanisms (Muscle & Fitness, 2024). A structured Adaptive Performance State (APS) process helps athletes recognize stress triggers, identify effective coping mechanisms, and transfer mental strategies into high-pressure situations.

One of the key functions of APS is to optimize the balance between the Sympathetic Nervous System (SNS), which triggers the body's *"fight or flight"* response, and the Parasympathetic Nervous System (PNS), which promotes relaxation through its "rest and digest" functions. High-pressure situations often lead to SNS over-activation, resulting in increased heart rate, muscle tension, and anxiety. However, a structured APS process enables athletes to regulate these responses through mental and physiological adaptation (Ben Foodman, 2024).

A key component of APS is goal setting. Goal setting helps athletes align their focus with a clear purpose, creating clarity and agency while helping manage anxiety. By setting achievable objectives, athletes create a roadmap that provides direction and stability in high-pressure moments. For example, a basketball player at the free-throw line can maintain composure by recalling a pre-set goal of following a consistent shooting rhythm (Applied Sport Psychology, n.d.).

In addition to goal setting, awareness of stress responses allows athletes to manage their emotional state effectively. Through self-monitoring, they can recognize when anxiety is rising and apply relaxation techniques such as deep breathing to regain focus. A tennis player, for instance, who becomes frustrated after an unforced error can use controlled breathing to reset their mindset before the next point (Halson, 2014).

Skill development is another crucial aspect of APS, requiring athletes to accept challenges as part of growth. Viewing setbacks as learning opportunities rather than failures fosters mental resilience. A gymnast who embraces the learning process rather than fearing mistakes will be better equipped to handle nerves during competition (Stonewall Performance, 2023).

Cognitive restructuring is essential in APS because it helps athletes recognize negative thoughts and replace them with constructive self-talk. Instead of thinking, *"I can't afford to miss this shot,"* a soccer player can reframe their mindset with a positive statement like, *"I've practiced this countless times, I'm ready."* This shift reduces SNS activation and promotes confidence (Success Starts Within, 2023).

Mindfulness and relaxation techniques further support APS by activating the PNS and enhancing awareness and composure. Meditation, controlled breathing, and visualization are widely used strategies that reinforce composure. Many elite athletes, including Michael Phelps, have utilized visualization techniques to mentally rehearse performances, ensuring smoother execution under pressure (Frontiers for Young Minds, 2022).

Establishing pre-performance routines enhances an athlete's ability to apply mental strategies in real-world scenarios. A sprinter who follows the same warm-up sequence before every race creates a sense of consistency, which reinforces stability and minimizes stress-related performance dysfunctions (Sport Psychology Today, n.d.).

By consistently engaging in structured APS strategies, athletes develop the ability to adapt to various challenges while maintaining composure. Over time, these self-regulatory practices enhance mental resilience, allowing athletes to remain aware, composed, and aligned with their performance goals. This approach not only optimizes performance but also fosters long-term well-being, ensuring one is prepared to be in their ideal performance state. An individual in APS exhibits heightened situational awareness, emotional resilience, and cognitive flexibility. Physiological markers often associated with APS include balanced autonomic nervous system (ANS) regulation, efficient energy expenditure, and optimized neural activation patterns (e.g., appropriate brainwave activity for the task) (Frontiers in Psychology, 2023).

Lastly, it is essential to recognize and understand why one's Optimal Performance State (OPS) is highly context dependent. OPS for a PGA Tour player on the last hole of a major while tied for the lead is very different from an NFL lineman on a goal-line play in the Super Bowl. Furthermore, neither of those OPS mindset frameworks is probably aligned with the appropriate mindset at a celebratory dinner with your partner, family, and friends. This further illustrates the importance of thought management via the APS process (Canadian Sport Institute Pacific, 2006).

How can athletes work on their self-belief?
- Every day; by recognizing and reframing
negative thoughts and feelings.
- Every day; by identifying and practicing
adaptive strategies.
- Every day; by aligning with and learning from
those of similar ethos and character.
- Every day; through intentions and actions
aligned with personal values.
- Every day; by training skill competencies and
mindset through imagery with absolute clarity.
Why? Because if it's truly important to you, you
will find a way.

CHAPTER 14

Why Routines Are So Important

A well-structured routine plays a pivotal role in enhancing neuroplasticity, which refers to the brain's capacity to reorganize itself by forming new neural connections throughout life. One effective method to promote neuroplasticity is the APS structured process, a sequence designed to bridge the gap between intention and outcome. Whether used in its original form or tailored to meet individual needs, APS serves as a system to manage the adaptive processes that lead to success. By following a consistent and repeatable routine, individuals improve the likelihood of achieving predictable, positive outcomes across various areas of life.

The primary benefit of a structured routine is consistency. A routine offers a stable environment that reinforces learning and habit formation. Engaging in the same activity repeatedly signals the brain to strengthen the neural pathways related to that behavior, making performance smoother over time. This consistency creates a foundation for long-term success by promoting the reinforcement of learned skills and behaviors (Schwartz, 2023).

Another critical benefit is the promotion of focused attention. Structured routines help minimize distractions and enhance concentration, which are essential for effective learning. This focused attention allows the brain to adapt and reorganize itself in response to new information, a crucial component of neuroplasticity. By concentrating on a specific task or skill, individuals optimize their capacity to form new brain connections (Pascual-Leone et al., 2015).

Incremental challenges within a structured routine also play a significant role in enhancing neuroplasticity. Gradually increasing the difficulty or complexity of tasks stimulates the brain and encourages adaptation. This progressive challenge prompts the brain to reorganize, facilitating growth and the formation of new neural pathways. This method of continuous adaptation is vital for promoting long-term cognitive development and maintaining brain plasticity (Klingberg, 2018). There is no better example of this than Earl Woods bringing distractions into Tiger Woods's performance routine during training, just as Richard Williams and Nick Bollettieri did with Serena and Venus Williams.

Additionally, a structured routine helps reinforce new skills. Consistently practicing new behaviors or abilities is essential for solidifying neural changes in the brain. A well-designed routine allows individuals to engage regularly in activities that reinforce new patterns, ensuring these behaviors become deeply ingrained over time. This regular practice strengthens the neural pathways required for the long-term formation of habits (Bezzina & Rollo, 2022).

In conclusion, a structured routine creates an environment that supports neuroplasticity by providing consistency, focused attention, incremental challenges, stress reduction, multisensory learning, and feedback loops. These components work together to enhance the brain's ability to reorganize itself, resulting in the formation of new neural connections and successful outcomes. Additionally, a structured routine is vital during the self-regulation phase of the APS construct, helping athletes manage both internal and external challenges at all levels, which promotes not only performance but also overall well-being.

CHAPTER 15

Self-Regulation

One's ability to self-regulate is a key component of the APS construct, as it enables athletes to manage their thoughts, emotions, and behaviors to optimize performance and well-being.

APS operates across four key domains:

- Cognitive Regulation: Conscious monitoring and directing of thoughts. In APS, thinking becomes purposeful, strategic, and adaptive rather than reactive.
- Emotional Regulation: Management of emotional intensity and valence. APS allows individuals to stay composed under pressure and avoid emotional hijacking (Gross, 2015).
- Behavioral Regulation: Alignment of actions with intentions. In APS, behaviors are executed deliberately, not impulsively.
- Physiological Regulation: Maintenance of optimal arousal levels through techniques including breath control, postural awareness, and energy regulation (Thompson et al., 2022).

Each domain contributes synergistically to achieving the desired Adaptive Performance State. The process begins with self-awareness, followed by monitoring and adjusting internal states in response to both internal and external challenges, thereby increasing the likelihood of consistent high-level performance under pressure. Every phase of the APS framework supports athletes in managing stress, fatigue, and external factors, while enhancing their ability to regulate emotions and physiological states, key self-regulatory tasks necessary for thriving.

The first stage, recognition, involves becoming aware of emotional and physiological states that may affect performance, such as stress, anxiety, or fatigue. Wearable technologies, including heart rate monitors and Body Battery metrics, help athletes track their energy levels and stress, providing real-time feedback that supports recognizing entry into less optimal states (Herold et al., 2019).

Once awareness is established, the next step is to identify the source of discomfort, whether it is simply fatigue, travel strain, environmental changes, or personal stressors. Emotional regulation becomes essential here, enabling athletes to distinguish between controllable and uncontrollable factors. Recognizing these triggers enables the application of effective coping strategies (Baumeister & Vohs, 2016).

The third stage, alignment, involves aligning mindset, the present objective, and actions with the demands of the moment. This stage ensures athletes are mentally and emotionally primed for action. Techniques such as positive self-talk, relaxation, and cognitive reframing help adjust focus and emotion. Wearables offer additional support here by providing biofeedback on stress levels and physiological conditions, helping athletes synchronize physical readiness with performance energy demands.

Transfer, the next phase, focuses on applying strategies learned from training in real-world, often more intense competition settings. Whether in unfamiliar venues or under different conditions, transferring emotional and physiological regulation skills is essential. Wearable data can track the effectiveness of coping strategies, informing adjustments during a performance.

Acceptance is the final stage. It involves acknowledging and embracing inevitable challenges, such as jet lag, fatigue, or adverse weather, and responding with adaptability. This mindset encourages athletes to focus on what can be controlled while letting go of what cannot. Techniques like mindfulness reinforce this resilience, supporting emotional balance even in the face of adversity (Kabat-Zinn, 2005).

Today, wearable technology plays an increasingly important role in supporting self-regulation. Devices track stress, heart rate variability, and Body Battery levels, providing insights that athletes can use to adjust in real-time. These tools inform decisions regarding hydration, nutrition, recovery, relaxation, and sleep, all of which are vital to adapting performance strategies on the go.

Travel-related fatigue is a significant factor in self-regulation. Crossing time zones can disrupt circadian rhythms, leading to poor sleep and reduced performance. Similarly, environmental stressors like heat, humidity, or altitude require heightened awareness and proactive recovery management. Recognizing early signs of fatigue and adjusting accordingly is critical. Prioritizing sleep quality, proper hydration, nutrition, and restorative practices helps maintain physiological balance.

In conclusion, self-regulation is a foundational skill for athletes aiming to achieve consistent, high-level performance. Through the APS framework, individuals can manage both emotional and physiological responses more effectively. Although athletes have performed without wearable technology for generations, modern tools provide new layers of awareness, offering real-time insights that enhance decision-making, adaptation, resilience, and well-being.

*"**Clutch State**" refers to a performance state experienced during high-pressure, challenging situations where success depends on quick, adaptive, and intuitive skills. Unlike "**flow,**" which involves effortless, automatic performance, clutch performance is marked by recognition, decisive action, alignment with the task, and heightened awareness of the context.*

CHAPTER 16

Stress and Anxiety in Athletic Performance

Stress and anxiety are related yet distinct concepts that significantly influence athletic performance and psychological well-being. Stress refers to the body's natural response to external challenges or demands, referred to as stressors, and can manifest as either eustress (positive stress) or distress (negative stress) depending on the context (Selye, 1974). Common stressors in athletics include competition, training demands, environmental factors, and personal life events. These stressors activate the sympathetic nervous system, triggering physiological changes such as increased heart rate, elevated muscle tension, and heightened sensory alertness (McEwen, 1998). These changes can enhance focus and performance in high-pressure situations when effectively managed.

In contrast, anxiety is characterized by a more persistent state of apprehension or worry, often disconnected from a specific external stimulus (American Psychiatric Association, 2022). Anxiety tends to revolve around perceived threats or uncontrollable outcomes and is more likely to disrupt concentration, impair motor control, and diminish confidence (Martens et al., 1990). While stress can be adaptive in performance settings, excessive or unmanaged anxiety often leads to negative performance outcomes and can even contribute to burnout if left unaddressed.

Understanding the distinction between stress and anxiety is vital for selecting appropriate intervention strategies. For instance, acute stress can often be redirected positively through visualization and focus enhancement techniques (Vealey & Chase, 2016). In contrast, managing anxiety may require deeper emotional regulation tools such as diaphragmatic breathing, mindfulness practices, or cognitive-behavioral interventions (Gross, 2015). Athletes who can distinguish between the two are better positioned to develop individualized mental performance strategies.

Moreover, effectively managing stress and anxiety within the APS framework equips athletes with transferable life skills. Coping strategies refined in sports environments can be applied in personal and professional domains, enhancing overall emotional resilience. Chronic anxiety, however, may require long-term psychological support and potential clinical intervention beyond basic sports psychology tools.

Ultimately, learning to identify and manage stress and anxiety is a foundational component of long-term mental health and performance sustainability. Rather than attempting to eliminate these experiences, athletes are encouraged to embrace them as part of the competitive landscape and develop skills that allow them to remain composed, present, and adaptive under pressure.

CHAPTER 17

Composure

Emotional composure refers to one's ability to regulate emotions and maintain a calm, collected state of mind, even in the face of challenging or stressful situations. It is not about suppressing emotions or feigning indifference. Rather, it involves acknowledging emotions and choosing how to respond, rather than simply reacting to them. This skill is fundamental in the decision-making process (intention) and plays a critical role in determining one's behavior and performance in both sports and life.

Remaining composed, especially when dealing with anxiety, is essential for achieving optimal performance. The following strategies can help maintain composure and shift perspective during anxious moments. These tools can be used to stay calm before a performance or as a reset during stressful triggers. Composure starts with awareness:

- Set the intention of achieving your Ideal Performance State. Recognize and train with resilience, composure, and acceptance so that these attributes become default actions under pressure.
- Engage in calm, positive self-talk; visualize *"green file"* shots. Ask questions like, *"Is my priority to influence my technique or the golf ball?"*
- Practice box breathing. 4 secs in, 4 secs hold, 4 secs out, 4 secs hold. It can be combined with mindful nature observation.
- Use positive imagery: Visualize successful shots while mimicking the feel using your open trail hand. Imagine performing with calm confidence.

- Rehearse your pre-shot routine using positive body language. Play the shot in your mind before executing it.

- Use positive word cues such as *"confident,"* *"trust,"* *"feel,"* or *"ready"* to stay grounded, especially when negotiating with the inner critic (Gould et al., 2002).

- Light physical activity, such as arm swings, walking, or stretching, helps relieve tension and reduce intrusive thoughts.

- Accept adversity as part of the game. Control your response rather than expecting perfection. Neutral self-talk can redirect your attention back to the present.

- Revisit journal notes from a day with an outcome you'd like to replicate.

- When doubt arises, ask questions that invite positive answers, e.g., *"Am I prepared?" "Am I ready?"*

- Use Progressive Muscle Relaxation (PMR): Tense a muscle group to a 10, hold for 4 seconds, then release to a 2 (Jacobson, 1938).

- Create a performance mantra aligned with your values. Repeated use strengthens presence and resilience. Examples: *"Embrace the challenge," "Trust my training,"* or *"I love this stuff."*

- Apply anchoring techniques: Use physical cues (e.g., touching thumb and forefinger) to cue a return to composure. Again, slow, deep breathwork can assist in this process.

- Recognize when triggered (e.g., anger). Like anxiety or self-doubt, recognizing the state is key. The APS process involves pausing, accepting, acknowledging, responding, and moving on. Follow your personal rules, three steps, 10 seconds, or one breathing cycle, to reset.

- Mantras can support goal focus, mental rehearsal, and presence by discouraging rumination on past/future outcomes.

- Cultivate gratitude. Be thankful for your skill, preparation, and presence. Unresolved external issues can become distractions;

awareness and the ability to mentally *"change the channel"* are essential to sustaining an adaptive state.

Incorporating these techniques into regular practice can significantly enhance emotional regulation, helping athletes perform with greater consistency, calmness, and clarity.

When we become truly aware, we lessen our dependence on negative thought patterns and behaviors. As our capacity outweighs our load, we overcome fear rather than letting it control us.

CHAPTER 18

Sensory Focus

Within the scope of APS, particularly in the context of golf, focus plays a crucial role. Understanding the functional differences between focal, thought, and temporal focus can help one recognize "what's important now" and enhance their preparation and execution (Weinberg & Gould, 2019).

Focal focus involves concentrating on specific cues relevant to the task, such as the ball, start line, shot shape, or technique if focusing on swing mechanics. Before executing a shot, golfers can use focal focus to identify key aspects of their performance. For example, a golfer might concentrate on the ball position in their stance, then focus on a landing area or intermediate target. This helps reduce distractions and improve concentration during practice and competition (Moran, 2016).

Thought focus involves directing one's attention toward cognitive processes, such as a conscious strategic "feel" cue activation, or self-talk. This type of focus addresses what one is thinking about during the pre-shot phase of the performance routine. During this phase, thoughts must align with the desired outcome, remain constructive, and promote confidence (Gardner & Moore, 2007). Recognizing unhelpful thoughts and transferring them into positive or neutral ones enhances mental readiness (Beilock, 2010).

Temporal focus refers to a focus on the sequencing and timing of actions. These include actions such as maintaining a swing tempo, achieving body balance, adjusting club position within the swing (during drills or rehearsals performed at significantly slower speed than "performance" speed), and/or timing focus breathing before executing a shot or reframing a moment of doubt. Establishing a repeatable routine aligns one's mental and physical processes, creating a structured rhythm that enhances stability (Cotterill, 2010).

Effective preparation in golf often requires the integration of all three types of focus:

- **Focal focus** eliminates distractions by concentrating on immediate targets and framing the current shot.
- **Thought focus** fosters a positive mindset, strengthens strategic thinking, and builds trust, which is essential for calming the prefrontal cortex's urge to control the swing during execution (Beilock, 2010).
- **Temporal focus** raises the probability that actions are fluid, synchronizing timing and movement for peak performance (Jackson & Csikszentmihalyi, 1999).

Sensory focus becomes a key part of meta-awareness when you intentionally recognize that you are paying attention to a specific sensory experience. In this case, meta-awareness observes and reflects on the act of sensory attention itself, rather than just being absorbed in it (Lutz et al., 2008). Sensory focus involves deliberately directing attention to sensory input, such as sights, sounds, and physical sensations, without negative judgment or interpretation. Instead of getting caught up in thoughts or emotions, one reverts to immediate experiences, like the sensation of breathing or the sights, sounds, and touches of the present environment (Kabat-Zinn, 2005).

As a bridge to meta-awareness, sensory focus helps athletes move beyond their usual thought patterns to observe their mental and emotional states, rather than being trapped by them. This process develops the ability to see thoughts as temporary events in the mind rather than absolute truths, laying a foundation for mindfulness (Gardner & Moore, 2007).

Functioning as a reframing tool, sensory focus interrupts cycles of negative thinking, which may include fear of failure, frustration, or self-criticism, by grounding attention in the neutral, present sensory experience. This shift creates psychological space, allowing the athlete to choose a more skillful response rather than reacting automatically (Moore & Gardner, 2011).

The significance of sensory focus for a mindful athlete is substantial; it boosts resilience, enhances attention under pressure, reduces performance anxiety, and helps maintain flow states by grounding awareness in the present, rather than getting caught up in stories about the past or future. (Jackson & Csikszentmihalyi, 1999; Kabat-Zinn, 2005).

Within the APS framework, the goal is to develop a highly aware, responsive, and efficient mind-body state that aligns with the demands of the situational challenge.

A Physical Cue

Much like the open trail hand rehearsal of face and path into, and exiting imaginary impact within the golf pre-shot rehearsal, the thumb-forefinger sensory connection serves as both a neurological and attentional gateway into APS for several reasons.

- **Triggering Self-Regulation:** The act of forming the thumb-forefinger connection physically cues the brain to transition towards centeredness, moving away from stress, distraction, or over-arousal, and into a regulated performance state (Siegel, 2020).

- **Enhancing Interoceptive Awareness:** The subtle tactile feedback heightens awareness of internal bodily states, such as heartbeat, breath, and muscle tone, which are critical cues in recognizing and sustaining APS (Craig, 2002).
- **Anchoring Present-Moment Focus:** APS necessitates dynamic present-moment awareness as opposed to reactive or distracted mindsets. The thumb-forefinger connection serves as a physical and mental anchor for attention, thereby strengthening this adaptive focus (Gardner & Moore, 2007).
- **Symbolizing Intentional Activation: This** connection can be employed as a ritualized "on-switch," functioning as a symbolic and neurological signal indicating a shift into intentional, adaptive action.
- **Facilitating Neuroplastic Reinforcement:** Through consistent repetition, the thumb-forefinger connection associates this simple gesture with entry into APS, subsequently strengthening neural pathways via practice and conditioning the brain for more rapid and seamless transitions into peak performance states (Doidge, 2007).

By consciously recognizing and activating these types of focus during both the non-routine and routine phases of one's APS cycle, one can recognize and align their mental state for greater consistency on the course. Additionally, incorporating drills that transfer these focusing techniques from practice to competition can solidify their effectiveness in high-pressure scenarios.

CHAPTER 19

Self-Talk

Self-talk is a vital component in an athlete's performance routines. It is the voice that leads an athlete's Adaptive Performance State. Neutral self-talk helps in reframing and refocusing, while positive self-talk boosts confidence and motivation. Recognizing negative self-talk enables athletes to strategically reframe these thoughts into more neutral ones (Hardy, 2006; Van Raalte et al., 2016).

Self-talk plays a vital role in one's mind management toolkit, significantly impacting an athlete's performance and mental well-being. Neutral self-talk serves as a foundation for reframing negative thoughts and refocusing attention, allowing athletes to recalibrate their mindset during high-pressure situations (Theodorakis et al., 2012).

Positive self-talk can also enhance an athlete's confidence and motivation, promoting a more positive outlook and improving performance (Hatzigeorgiadis et al., 2009). However, athletes must be able to identify instances of negative self-talk, as these harmful thoughts can hurt performance and self-esteem (Van Raalte et al., 1995).

By acknowledging and evaluating these negative patterns, athletes can strategically shift their self-dialogue from negative to neutral, creating a more constructive inner narrative that supports their goals and performance. This conscious effort to reframe self-talk not only helps in managing stress but also cultivates resilience and focus, essential traits for success in sports (Hardy, 2006; Latinjak et al., 2017).

Personal culture is a reflection of our actions, not our words. Our actions define who we really are. Act accordingly.

CHAPTER 20

Managing Perception

The APS construct of Recognize, Identify, Align, Adapt, and Accept provides a straightforward framework for athletes to manage their decisions and behavior, particularly during times when they are influenced by perception or facing challenging situations (Gardner & Moore, 2007; Vealey, 2007).

First, athletes recognize the emerging emotions, thoughts, and perceptions, acknowledging and accepting their mental state. This awareness enables them to differentiate between feelings and actions, or to determine whether the perceived threat is real or not (Gross, 2015). Next, one must identify the source of emotions or thoughts, which helps them determine whether their perception is based on a previous experience or simply a negative bias towards the current challenge (Beilock, 2010; Lazarus, 2000).

Following identification, the athlete works to align their thoughts, emotions, and actions with their goals, focusing on reframing their mindset to remain opportunistic and solution-oriented (Moore, 2009). The athlete is now in an adaptive state, rather than a reactive state, and is better prepared to adjust their strategies or mindset as needed to respond to the current situation with flexibility (Kashdan & Rottenberg, 2010).

Finally, acceptance allows the athlete to recognize the outcome, regardless of the result, without resistance, but with clarity for what it is: a moment, successful or otherwise. This reduces the impact of perceived failure and facilitates quicker recovery (Hayes et al., 2006; Gardner & Moore, 2012). The APS sequence helps athletes maintain a higher level of recognition over their perceptions and navigate challenges in a mentally resilient manner, optimizing both mental and physical performance (Birrer & Morgan, 2010).

CHAPTER 21

Accepting Change

The APS framework supports change by guiding individuals through a structured process of skill learning, understanding, and application, which enhances brain flexibility to accept new pathways. This process involves forming new neural connections and reorganizing existing pathways, enabling athletes to improve their skills and optimize their movements (Kolb & Gibb, 2011; Thomas & Baker, 2021). In sports, three key elements, awareness, alignment, and skill transfer, are greatly influenced by the APS model.

Awareness is essential for athletes as it enables them to recognize their body movements and understand their positioning in space. By engaging in mindful practices and feedback mechanisms, athletes can cultivate a heightened sense of awareness through neural pathway changes in the brain (Tang et al., 2015; Schmeichel & Tang, 2015). This improved awareness can lead to better decision-making and responsiveness in all phases of athletic development and life.

In the context of accepting change, recognition encourages individuals to become aware of their existing skills and knowledge, serving as a foundation for growth. Identifying areas where changes or improvements are needed promotes targeted learning and a *"periodized"* plan of progression from skill acquisition to skill application (Bompa & Buzzichelli, 2019). Aligning one's mindset and actions to ensure they are in sync with new insights or challenges allows for a cohesive learning experience.

Skill transfer emphasizes the application of newly acquired skills in different contexts, reinforcing the neural pathways associated with those skills (Barnett & Ceci, 2002). Lastly, acceptance fosters an open mindset toward change and adaptation, which is crucial for embracing new experiences, changes, or perceived threats (Crane et al., 2019). Together, these elements create a comprehensive framework that not only supports personal and professional growth but also stimulates the brain's ability to reorganize and develop, underscoring the importance of adaptability in learning and performance (Davidson & Begley, 2012).

CHAPTER 22

Overcoming Negative Projections

Young athletes frequently face avoidance-based thinking, particularly when they focus on potential negative outcomes. Utilizing APS strategies can help them reframe their resistance and navigate these challenges effectively (Beilock, 2010; Weinberg & Gould, 2019).

The first step is to recognize avoidance behaviors caused by perception rather than reality and understand their negative impact on performance. Athletes should be encouraged to reflect on situations where fear of failure or negative judgment causes hesitation or withdrawal (Conroy & Metzler, 2004). Recognizing these patterns is essential for initiating change; often, these negative thoughts are prompted not by actual circumstances but by reactions to unknown factors, such as the uncertainties that come with a new environment or facing a larger, seemingly more formidable opponent (Jones et al., 2002).

After identifying avoidance behaviors and negative thoughts, athletes need to determine specific triggers that cause these reactions. This involves recognizing specific stress-inducing situations, tasks, or thoughts that lead to anxiety or fear. For example, an athlete may experience increased stress during high-stakes competitions or when attempting complex skills (Martinent & Ferrand, 2006). Recognizing these triggers helps develop targeted interventions. Once a negative trigger is identified, the next step is to match coping strategies to effectively manage it. Strategies include cognitive restructuring, which involves challenging and reframing negative thoughts to foster a more positive and realistic mindset (Beck, 2011; Hanton et al., 2005). Adjusting goals, especially unrealistic expectations, involves setting more attainable, process-oriented objectives that focus on performance processes, skill mastery, or personal development rather than solely focusing on outcomes (Dweck, 2006).

Additionally, developing or refining performance routines, which encompass pre-performance, performance, and post-performance routines, is essential. Establishing consistent routines prior to performance helps foster predictability and alleviate anxiety (Cotterill, 2010). This structured approach enables athletes to confront avoidance-based thinking, mitigate the impact of negative outcome anticipations, and enhance both their athletic performance and personal growth.

Engaging in deep breathing, meditation, or progressive muscle relaxation can help manage arousal levels, while reframing techniques enable athletes to shift their perspectives and apply critical thinking skills more effectively, rather than merely reacting to the fear of failure (Gardner & Moore, 2007; Gross, 2015).

The final step involves transferring the coping strategies learned in sports to other areas of life, thereby enhancing overall resilience. By applying these skills, which range from imagery to practice within their competitive environments, athletes can more effectively manage academic pressures, social challenges such as conformity pressure, and performance-related stressors (Gucciardi et al., 2009).

CHAPTER 23

Task Transfer & Orientation

Within the APS framework, task orientation refers to an athlete's current focus or intention, whether it is technical development, skill improvement, or performance. In contrast, task transfer involves applying skills learned in one context, such as strategic planning, to another, like rehearsal, or from rehearsal to action, or even from one sport to another (Barnett & Ceci, 2002; Magill & Anderson, 2017). Both are vital for performance and well-being; recognizing the specific focus at the moment helps an athlete decide which task process needs attention. Task orientation increases motivation and resilience, while task transfer allows athletes to adapt quickly to new challenges and environments (Dweck, 2006; Roberts et al., 2007).

Effectively aligned, task orientation and task transfer are both essential in developing an athlete's cognitive and performance adaptive skills. Task orientation refers to an athlete's internal motivation to improve, emphasizing effort, learning, and mastery rather than external validation or comparison with others (Nicholls, 1989; Ames, 1992).

This mindset encourages long-term resilience, adaptability, and steady performance growth (Roberts, 2012). Task transfer, however, involves applying learned skills to different tasks within one's chosen sport(s) and/or life skills, thereby increasing versatility and problem-solving (Perkins & Salomon, 1992). For example, a basketball player with strong footwork might successfully transfer that skill to soccer, improving agility and coordination. Together, these concepts shape an athlete's mental adaptability, helping them stay engaged, develop well-rounded abilities, and maximize performance across various challenges (Gould & Voelker, 2012).

Task Transfer: The bridge from Intention to Action

At its core, the function of task transfer is the ability to apply APS tools and seamlessly transition from one present-moment focus to the next without being distracted by internal or external noise. Within the Adaptive Performance State (APS) framework, task transfer signifies the critical transition between cognitive intent and embodied execution. It takes place in the narrow bandwidth that connects the information-gathering and movement phases, where perception turns into action.

Specifically, in the case of an elite golfer's pre-shot routine, this transition occurs through three clearly connected steps: target acquisition, pattern rehearsal, and target reorientation, complemented by focused breathing and a deliberate walk-in. Each step acts as a cognitive-to-kinesthetic bridge, ensuring that actions are most likely to match intent through clear sensory registration, precise motor recruitment, and continuous adaptive focus.

1. Target Acquisition: The Neural Anchor of Intent

High-quality sensory input promotes high-quality motor activation. During the framing phase, target acquisition acts as the neural anchor that stabilizes the system for optimal performance. The golfer's perceptual field narrows as they deliberately focus on visual and spatial details, such as the contrasts, colors, and contours of the target environment. This focused attention activates the prefrontal cortex (PFC) for organized attention while also preparing the spatial mapping, distance calibration, and target registration.

Crucially, this is not a passive act of *"looking."* It is the act of knowing, of embedding intention into perception. Clarity of target detail leads to clarity of purpose; clarity of purpose stabilizes confidence. Through this, trust begins to form as a neurocognitive state, an internal coherence between sensory input and motor expectation. When the golfer recognizes that the true target is the start line, not the final destination, perceptual depth is reframed toward process rather than outcome, maintaining PFC engagement while reducing external cognitive noise.

2. Pattern Rehearsal: Encoding the Motor Map

Once the target is precisely encoded, the pattern rehearsal stage integrates the cognitive plan with the body's motor schema. Here, the golfer moves from perceptual registration to motor simulation, the brain's internal rehearsal of action sequences that mirror the intended shot. Neural efficiency is maximized when this rehearsal reflects both the strategic plan and the emotional tone of commitment.

Within the APS model, pattern rehearsal functions as the motor priming mechanism that indicates readiness for transfer. The sensory and visual clarity established through framing now guides the body's preparatory networks. The motor cortex, cerebellum, and basal ganglia synchronize via predictive coding, simulating the desired movement pattern before physical execution. Any discrepancy between the perceived target data and motor intention is detected and adjusted in real-time. When alignment occurs, with the brain's internal model matching the external target representation, confidence shifts from a concept to a state of readiness.

3. Target Reorientation, Focused Breath, and Walk-In: Transfer

The final stage of task transfer, which includes target reorientation, focused breathing, and walking in, marks the release of cognitive control and the start of adaptive flow. After rehearsal, the golfer visually and mentally returns to the target to confirm spatial registration and emotional stability. This brief reorientation acts as a synchronization cue, aligning perception, intention, and motor memory.

The focused breath that follows serves two functions: physiological regulation and neural recalibration. It reduces cortical dominance, lowers PFC interference, and initiates a parasympathetic calming response. This decrease in cognitive noise facilitates the transition from explicit control to implicit execution, a key shift that defines the APS's movement from deliberate thinking to intuitive action.

The walk-in sequence becomes a rhythmic expression of commitment. Each step symbolizes transforming abstract intent into confident movement founded on trust. The movement cue indicates shifting from prefrontal-driven thinking to subcortical–sensorimotor readiness. At this moment, the golfer's system fully synchronizes, with sensory input, motor preparedness, and emotional stability aligned toward a single goal: an action that reflects their intention.

A Cohesive Flow

The linkage between these steps is not mechanical but rather a cohesive flow. Each stage feeds the next through coherent neurocognitive communication:

- Clear sensory framing primes confident motor mapping.
- Accurate rehearsal stabilizes the sensorimotor network for execution.
- Intentional reorientation and breath regulate arousal, securing transition into automatic flow.

When this sequence remains uninterrupted, task transfer within the APS framework indicates a smooth handover of control from conscious thought to subconscious execution. In this context, the elite golfer's pre-shot routine becomes a seamless transition from prefrontal-dependent thinking to subcortical–sensorimotor execution (swing motion triggered by the movement cue), which enhances the likelihood of actions matching the intent. Essentially, procedural memory is the long-term, non-declarative storage of motor skills, and its formation and execution fundamentally rely on specific subcortical sensorimotor loops that become more highly efficient through practice.

The Concept of Adaptive Performance State Flow Chart

Stable confidence emerges when one learns to recognize what's happening internally, identify the trigger or pattern, align with desired behavior or intent, Transfer focus back to the task, and accept the outcome as feedback, not failure.

CHAPTER 24

Reframing

Reframing is a cognitive approach that helps athletes recognize their perceptions of situations, events, or experiences. It often shifts an opposing or unproductive viewpoint into a more positive or constructive one, enabling an athlete to navigate around an obstacle rather than freeze or operate with a fear-based mindset (Weinberg & Gould, 2019).

A primary use of reframing is in alleviating performance anxiety. Athletes frequently face anxiety before major events, spurred by the pressures to succeed or fears of failing. By reframing their thoughts, they can shift their viewpoint from perceiving the situation as a threat to viewing it as a challenge or an opportunity for growth (Jones, 1995). For instance, an athlete may reframe their mindset from "I must win this match to avoid disappointing everyone" to *"This is an opportunity to test my skills and grow, irrespective of the result."*

Moreover, reframing plays a vital role in building confidence. Athletes can view setbacks, such as missing a shot or losing a game, as learning opportunities instead of failures. This process fosters resilience by encouraging athletes to consider mistakes as integral to their improvement (Sarkar & Fletcher, 2014). For example, a golfer who misses a key putt might reframe their thoughts from *"I ruined our chance to win"* to "Statistics show that a 7-foot putt has a 50% success rate on the PGA Tour, so let's remain positive and stick to our strategy for the next shot."

Reframing also sharpens focus by helping athletes concentrate on what they can manage. If external distractions arise, such as an opponent's assertive play or unfavorable weather, reframing helps them identify their controllable responses and adjust their focus accordingly (Hardy et al., 1996).

Another advantage of reframing is its role in encouraging positive self-talk. Negative internal dialogues, like *"I can't do this,"* can hinder performance. Reframing allows athletes to shift their mindset to a more empowering stance. Rather than thinking, *"I can't do this,"* an athlete might reframe that to, ***"I've successfully navigated tough situations before, and I can handle this"*** (Theodorakis et al., 2000).

During the reframing process, visualization and imagery prove essential as mental training techniques that enable athletes to rehearse skills and scenarios mentally without needing physical actions. These techniques engage various sensory inputs, primarily visual (observing performances), kinesthetic (sensing movement), and auditory (recognizing sounds such as a coach's commands or crowd noise), alongside specific motor skill cues and tactile experiences. By integrating these senses, athletes can create a vivid and realistic representation of performance scenarios, thus strengthening the neural pathways related to motor skills and better preparing them to adapt (Morris et al., 2005).

Imagery can be categorized into several types, including cognitive-specific (practicing individual skills), cognitive-general (rehearsing strategies or routines), motivational-specific (visualizing goal achievement), motivational-general mastery (improving focus, confidence, and resilience), and motivational-general arousal (controlling emotions and energy) (Hall et al., 1998). When used effectively, these imagery types boost adaptive performance by increasing focus, lowering anxiety, building confidence, and maintaining motivation. For example, an athlete might mentally rehearse a pre-performance routine using cognitive-general imagery to promote consistency and calmness, or use motivational-specific imagery to stay motivated during long training sessions by imagining the satisfaction of seeing progress or mastering a skill, rather than fixating solely on the often-unrealistic goal of dominating the field.

To implement these techniques effectively, athletes should engage with imagery consistently in a structured way, ideally in an environment free of distractions, utilizing all pertinent senses while focusing on both the physical and emotional aspects of their performance. A beneficial approach is to blend imagery with deep breathing or relaxation techniques to simulate high-pressure scenarios while maintaining calmness. Mental performance coaches can tailor imagery scripts for specific contexts, helping athletes prepare for competitions and navigate challenges such as injuries, fatigue, or performance slumps (Vealey & Greenleaf, 2010). By embedding these visualization strategies, athletes can cultivate a resilient, focused, and adaptive mindset that enhances peak performance.

Lastly, reframing helps sustain motivation. During tough training or competitive phases, athletes might experience discouragement. Reframing can help them accept struggles as part of their growth journey and recognize the importance of their efforts. An athlete might reflect, "Even though I'm fatigued, I wouldn't want to be anywhere else; let's keep pushing forward!" (Weinberg & Gould, 2019).

By integrating reframing strategies into their mental toolkit, athletes can better align their emotional and cognitive responses to challenges, apply positive thinking strategies in their daily routines, and develop a more resilient mindset that enhances one's readiness, adaptability, and performance.

Awareness is the conduit from unconsciously incompetent to consciously incompetent

---

CHAPTER 25

Mindfulness Practice for Emotional Regulation

Mindfulness practice helps athletes regulate frustration and anxiety, which are common challenges in sports performance (Baltzell & Summers, 2017). One of the fundamental aspects of mindfulness is awareness of thoughts and emotions. This practice encourages athletes to recognize their internal states without being unrealistically critical, allowing them to identify moments of frustration or anxiety (Kabat-Zinn, 1990). By developing this awareness, athletes can transfer their focus to constructive responses before negative emotions escalate (Gardner & Moore, 2007).

Breathing techniques are another essential component of mindfulness, as they help calm the nervous system and reduce physiological symptoms of anxiety, such as a rapid heart rate or shallow breathing (Jerath et al., 2006). Through mindful breathing, athletes can align their physiological and mental states, regaining composure and sustaining focus (Thompson et al., 2011). Additionally, mindfulness emphasizes the importance of staying present, which helps athletes recognize distractions stemming from past mistakes or future concerns and refocus on the immediate task at hand (Segal et al., 2013).

Mindfulness also promotes acceptance, encouraging athletes to accept emotions, including frustration and setbacks, rather than resisting them (Hayes et al., 1999). This reduces the negative impact these emotions may have on performance, allowing for a quicker return to an optimal state of mind. As a result, mindfulness improves focus by enhancing attention and concentration, helping athletes align with their performance goals rather than becoming consumed by stressors or distractions (Moore, 2009).

Beyond emotional regulation, mindfulness fosters resilience by helping athletes transfer their perspective from frustration to learning. This shift strengthens their ability to bounce back from negative experiences, making them more mentally tough in the face of adversity (Josefsson et al., 2017). Additionally, mindfulness often incorporates visualization and mental rehearsal, techniques that prepare athletes for high-pressure situations and enhance confidence by reducing anxious anticipation (Birrer et al., 2012).

By integrating mindfulness training into their daily routines, athletes can enhance emotional regulation, improve recovery, and increase focus, ultimately improving their performance. Working with a coach or therapist can help further identify mindfulness techniques that align with individual needs, maximizing their effectiveness in high-stakes competitive environments (Gardner & Moore, 2012).

CHAPTER 26

The Importance of Sleep

While the APS construct might not directly serve as the main function of a healthy sleep routine, the structured cue words play a crucial role in guiding what a person chooses to pay attention to. To optimize athletic performance, recovery, and overall well-being, it is vital to activate the parasympathetic nervous system (PNS) while calming the sympathetic nervous system (SNS). The sympathetic nervous system manages the body's *"fight or flight"* response, often leading to stress and tension, whereas the parasympathetic system oversees the *"rest and digest"* state, encouraging relaxation, recovery, and mental clarity (McCorry, 2007). Achieving this balance can be achieved through various adaptive strategies, including breath work, sensory techniques, and mindfulness practices.

Breathing exercises are among the most effective methods for activating the PNS and calming the SNS. Deep, slow breathing stimulates the vagus nerve, which plays a key role in the parasympathetic response (Sakakibara et al., 2013). Diaphragmatic breathing, or belly breathing, involves taking slow, deep breaths into the diaphragm instead of shallow chest breaths. A simple technique involves inhaling for 4 seconds, holding the breath for 4 seconds, and exhaling for 4 seconds, which helps reset the nervous system and promote calmness. Box breathing, which includes inhaling, holding, exhaling, and pausing, also provides a structured rhythm that can help reduce anxiety and improve focus (Brown & Gerbarg, 2005). Similarly, the 4-7-8 breathing technique, where one inhales for 4 seconds, holds for 7 seconds, and exhales for 8 seconds, further aids relaxation and slows the heart rate (Weil, 2011).

Progressive Muscle Relaxation (PMR) is an effective technique where athletes systematically tense and then relax different muscle groups, signaling the brain to ease up. This method not only helps release physical tension but also assists in shifting the mind from stress to calm (Jacobson, 1938; Bernstein & Borkovec, 1973). In addition to breath work, creating a sensory-rich, calming environment can further activate the parasympathetic nervous system. Nature sounds, such as rain or ocean waves, have been shown to lower cortisol levels and promote tranquility, helping athletes focus without mental distractions (Alvarsson et al., 2010). Binaural beats, which utilize two distinct sound frequencies in each ear to produce a third, can also foster a meditative state conducive to relaxation (Wahbeh et al., 2007). Likewise, white noise or soft instrumental music provides a steady, calming background that reduces stress and prevents overstimulation (Thoma et al., 2013).

Visualization and guided imagery provide mental techniques to shift from a sympathetic to a parasympathetic state. By imagining calming scenes or recalling successful past performances, athletes can lower stress and foster a sense of calm and confidence (Taylor et al., 1998). Guided meditation, which often includes body scans and breathing exercises, enhances this relaxation process. Mindfulness practices, like body scanning or mindful walking, where individuals focus on bodily sensations and movements, effectively promote awareness and release tension held in the body, encouraging a transition into a more relaxed state (Kabat-Zinn, 1990).

Temperature regulation, whether through cold or warmth, can help modulate nervous system activity. Cold exposure, like ice baths and hot/cold showers, activates the parasympathetic system after intense exertion, reducing muscle soreness and aiding recovery (Bleakley & Davison, 2010). Conversely, warm baths or heating pads encourage relaxation by easing muscle tension and activating the calming effects of the parasympathetic nervous system (Lundgren et al., 2014).

Lastly, positive self-talk and cognitive reframing can significantly help calm the mind and shift the nervous system into a more restful state. By adopting positive affirmations and focusing on controllable aspects of performance, athletes can counteract stress and anxiety. Reframing negative thoughts and replacing them with constructive perspectives encourages a more focused and calm mental state (Beck, 2011; Hardy et al., 2001).

In conclusion, activating the parasympathetic nervous system and calming the sympathetic nervous system are essential for optimal athletic performance, overall well-being, and effective sleep/recovery. Through techniques such as breath work, sensory relaxation, mindfulness, and cognitive strategies (illustrated in Chapter 8), one can reduce stress, improve focus, and enhance recovery, ultimately fostering a balanced and healthy mind-body connection.

Action starts in the imagination with a clear intention. Change does not happen by chance; it must be intentional and pursued with awareness, discipline, and acceptance.

CHAPTER 27

Detachment

Detachment within the APS framework refers to an athlete's ability to separate themselves emotionally from outcome-focused pressures during competition, training, or, most importantly, when transitioning from these environments into their home life or social setting. This skill is crucial for sustained performance and mental well-being (Gardner & Moore, 2007). One of its primary benefits is emotional regulation, as detachment enables athletes to recognize overwhelming emotions and create a psychological distance from them (Gross, 2015). By doing so, they maintain composure and stay present in high-pressure situations (Moore, 2009).

The ability to detach also enhances performance by allowing athletes to concentrate solely on execution rather than being distracted by anxiety, fear of failure, or external pressures (Birrer & Morgan, 2010). When athletes align their focus with the process rather than the outcome, they perform with greater confidence and clarity (Mallett & Hanrahan, 2004). Detachment also plays a critical role in building grit, as it enables athletes to identify failures or setbacks as learning opportunities rather than sources of self-doubt (Duckworth et al., 2007). By transferring their energy toward future improvements rather than dwelling on past mistakes, they develop resilience and a growth-oriented mindset (Yeager & Dweck, 2012).

Furthermore, detachment supports objective assessment. Athletes who maintain emotional distance from their performance can accept constructive criticism more effectively, making necessary adjustments without being held back by negative self-perception (Anderson et al.,

2004). This skill to evaluate performance with a clear, rational perspective leads to more consistent improvement over time (Hays, 2009).

Beyond competition, detachment is essential for maintaining a balance between sport and personal life. Many athletes struggle with tying their identity solely to their athletic achievements, which can lead to emotional distress during setbacks or career transitions (Brewer et al., 1993). Developing detachment allows athletes to recognize their broader identity beyond sports, preventing burnout and promoting overall well-being (Gustafsson et al., 2011).

Techniques such as mindfulness, meditation, and cognitive reframing will help athletes cultivate detachment, ultimately benefiting both their relationships, mental health, and athletic performance (Gardner & Moore, 2012). By incorporating these strategies, athletes can sustain high-level performance while maintaining emotional stability.

CHAPTER 28

Quieting the Mind

The notion of a *"quiet mind"* refers to a mental state characterized by minimal inner dialogue and reduced cognitive interference, enabling athletes to perform with clarity, fluidity, and instinctive accuracy. It represents a mental environment where overthinking lessens, allowing natural movement to arise from confidence and concentration (Gardner & Moore, 2007). In this context, the Adaptive Performance State (APS) provides a comprehensive framework for understanding how the mind transitions from thought to action, enabling athletes to maintain a calm mind during their performance.

The first step in this journey is identity alignment, where the athlete's self-concept aligns with the demands of the moment. When athletes adopt the belief, ***"I am built for this moment,"*** their actions stem from assurance rather than doubt. This alignment reduces ego-driven thoughts and promotes psychological stability (Vealey, 2007). Next, the athlete enters a phase of awareness and acceptance, recognizing both internal feelings (such as nerves and tension) and external factors (like crowd noise and the opponent's behavior) without resistance. Acceptance lessens cognitive struggles, allowing emotions and distractions to pass without interrupting focus (Kabat-Zinn, 1990).

At this point, an intention cue becomes vital to trigger functional movement and link the athlete to the specific task. This cue often consists of a simple, task-focused phrase or image, such as *"smooth drive," "find the seam,"* or a *"mental snapshot"* of the desired movement, serving as a psychological trigger. It prepares the neuromuscular system for action, transforming intentional thought into physical movement (Beilock & Carr,

2001). This process signifies the movement from thought to action, engaging the athlete's training and procedural memory while bypassing slower analytical thinking (Masters & Maxwell, 2008).

The interplay between brainwave activity and a *"quiet mind"* is crucial for managing one's mindset and effectively performing motor skills, especially within the intention-action loop framework. Brainwave patterns, notably alpha and theta waves, correlate strongly with a calm, focused mental state frequently referred to as the *"quiet mind"* (Baer, 2003; Thompson & Thompson, 2003). This state features reduced cognitive noise, less internal dialogue, and increased awareness of the present, all vital for refined motor control and adaptive performance, especially under pressure.

In mind management, a quiet mind enhances emotional regulation and focus, essential for synchronizing mental intention with physical action. When the brain exhibits dominant alpha waves (8–12 Hz), it indicates a relaxed yet alert mental state, which improves sensorimotor integration and reduces the impact of overthinking (Hatfield et al., 2004). Theta waves (4–8 Hz), often associated with deep focus or meditation, further enhance access to intuitive and automatic processes critical for skilled motor performance (Gruzelier, 2014). These brainwave states foster an environment where the brain's executive functions can temporarily recede, allowing procedural memory and inherent skills to take over, often described as being "in the zone" (Csikszentmihalyi, 1990).

Adaptive skill deployment within the motor-intention loop depends on this neural efficiency. A quiet mind allows the central nervous system to quickly interpret sensory information and perform motor responses without the hindrance of conscious thought (Moore et al., 2012). This ability is particularly essential in fast-paced environments, such as sports or high-pressure decision-making situations, where timely execution and smooth movement are crucial. With diminished mental noise and a calm mind, motor plans align seamlessly with the intention behind an action, leading to smoother and more adaptive responses. Therefore, fostering a quiet mind through brainwave regulation and cognitive techniques is essential for mastering the intention-motor loop and achieving high-level performance in any skill-based task.

As movement begins, the final aspect of the APS framework, detail integration, comes into play. The athlete focuses selectively on cues relevant to performance while filtering out irrelevant information. They remain adaptable to real-time details, such as an opponent's timing or subtle environmental shifts, without losing their rhythm (Abernethy, 2001). This heightened focus on the present supports ongoing adaptation and reinforces the quiet mind, enabling the athlete to sustain a fluid performance state.

In conclusion, the APS framework facilitates the athlete's transition from cognitive readiness to instinctive execution. Through identity alignment, internal state management via acceptance, activation of intention cues, and integration of key details, the athlete enters a state of purposeful movement, characterized by a quiet mind, intentional action, and deep immersion in the task at hand.

When you sit quietly and reflect, what are you connecting with? Are you connecting to a pathway towards well-being, or are you focusing on anxiety-inducing perceptions?

CHAPTER 29

Creating a New Habit

The structured format of the APS process is key to developing good habits, which are essential for enhancing performance, consistency, and mental resilience. Changing an athlete's habits and default actions is best facilitated in small doses with a specific purpose. All changes must include an associated mindset adjustment to prevent previous well-worn habits from coming to the forefront of memory function. How we communicate, both internally and externally, reflects what we focus on. Ensure that the messages you send are relevant to achieving your immediate goals.

Athletes must initially acknowledge their current habits, both beneficial and detrimental, to understand their impact on performance. Traditional habits, for simplicity, can be attributed to what is termed the *"Old Brain,"* a concept that will be elaborated upon later. For instance, an athlete may observe recurring pre-game anxiety or irregular training routines. Following this recognition, the subsequent step is to identify specific behaviors that contribute to either success or failure. This process involves pinpointing triggers, responses, and outcomes. For example, a basketball player might determine that taking deep breaths before executing a free throw enhances accuracy, thereby establishing a beneficial habit worth maintaining. Nevertheless, this new habit is connected to its origin within the **"New Brain,"** which will be discussed in greater detail later in this document.

After identification, it is crucial to ensure alignment between habits and performance goals. Aligning behaviors with training, mental preparation, and daily routines ensures they support peak performance.

For example, an athlete aiming to improve endurance must align their physiological training schedule with proper mental preparation, resources, nutrition, sleep, and recovery. The final step is rehearsal, where repetition and practice solidify habits, making them automatic. Both mental and physical rehearsal help athletes perform under pressure without overthinking. A golfer who consistently visualizes and practices their swing will develop muscle memory, leading to improved performance.

Establishing good habits offers numerous benefits. It promotes consistency, reducing performance fluctuations caused by external distractions or changes in mood. It also builds confidence, as athletes can rely on well-formed routines in competition. Additionally, structured habits help reduce anxiety, providing a sense of control, while also improving focus by streamlining decision-making. Moreover, maintaining proper training and recovery habits aids in injury prevention, ultimately prolonging an athlete's career.

A structured, systematic progression benefits decision-making by providing a clear framework that enhances the recognition of key patterns, trends, and potential risks, allowing for more accurate assessments. This structured approach strengthens commitment to a new habit by aligning decisions with well-defined objectives, reducing uncertainty, and increasing accountability. Furthermore, it fosters adaptive performance advantages by enabling continuous learning, refinement of strategies, and the ability to adjust to dynamic circumstances, ensuring resilience in applying one's new habits and achieving long-term success.

One significant point of clarity for young athletes and their parents regarding the often-misconceived notion that a habit (neural pathway) equals complete skill acquisition (mastery) is that this is not the case. A habit results from approximately 66 days of continuous practice (Lally et al., 2010). Mastery, on the other hand, requires 10,000 hours of dedicated work. These represent two very different levels of adaptation. Recognizing this fact is crucial for setting goals and for parents to have realistic expectations of their young athlete's performance capabilities, as well as for understanding the concept of *"muscle memory."* This term is frequently misused and misunderstood.

Again, while muscles themselves do not have memory, the concept of *"muscle memory"* refers to the brain's ability to automate motor movements through repetition and practice, leading to more efficient execution of physical tasks. While muscles do not have memory, the brain forms and strengthens neural pathways in areas such as the prefrontal cortex, basal ganglia, and cerebellum, which are responsible for planning, refining, and coordinating movement (Stanford Medicine, 2022). As these neural connections become more established, movements that were once structured, deliberate, and conscious gradually become automatic. This allows athletes to perform complex actions, such as a golf swing, a basketball free throw, or a gymnast's routine, with minimal conscious thought, once a strategic plan is in place. Feedback from the body, including sensory input from muscles and joints, also helps the brain adjust and refine movement patterns, further enhancing the automaticity and precision of the skill. Ultimately, *"muscle memory"* underscores the connection between the mind and body, as the brain stores and refines motor skills that the body executes with increasing efficiency over time.

Movement patterns, such as a golf swing, are encoded in the brain as part of motor memory, which involves a coordinated network of regions tasked with planning, executing, and refining movements. The motor cortex plays a central role in controlling voluntary muscle activity, whereas the cerebellum is crucial for ensuring proper timing, coordination, and balance. With repeated practice, the basal ganglia facilitate the transition from a swing to a more automatic and habitual action (Caligiore et al., 2017). Furthermore, the premotor cortex and supplementary motor area are essential for planning and sequencing the swing, while the somatosensory cortex provides feedback from muscles and joints, enabling real-time adjustments. These adjustments, as discussed earlier, are recognized during drills and rehearsals (modelling), not during competition. Any attempt to make real-time adjustments once a golf swing is in motion, in the act of hitting a golf shot, will interfere with one's ability to *"free swing"*. Through continuous practice, these brain regions work together more efficiently, resulting in the golf swing becoming increasingly fluid and natural over time, a phenomenon referred to as motor learning.

This awareness, connection, and acceptance can significantly influence the relationship between a young athlete's learning, motivation, and passion for their sport, as well as the relationship between parents and their young athlete. Unrealistic expectations are a significant reason why a young athlete may lose interest in sports and eventually quit.

CHAPTER 30

Physical Anchoring for Connection

Physical anchoring is the key to transferring, within the Adaptive Performance State (APS), it's the powerful connection between the body and the mind in optimizing performance, especially in high-pressure situations. Essentially, a physical anchor serves as a mechanism (action) that bridges the gap between the mind's control processes and the instinctual, feel-based motor skills that are necessary for the desired unencumbered motion that best serves one's performance needs.

The following is a breakdown of why a physical anchor is a key tool in the effective utilization of the APS process:

- **Pre-Frontal Cortex Control:** The prefrontal cortex is responsible for higher-order cognitive functions like decision-making, problem-solving, and exerting conscious control over our actions. In high-stakes or pressure-filled scenarios, the prefrontal cortex tends to become overactive, leading to overthinking, doubt, and even paralysis by analysis. This overactivation can hinder athletic performance because natural, fluid movement is often inhibited by the mind's need to control and assess every action (Lee, 2013; Williams, 2024).

- **Physical Anchoring as a Bridge:** A physical anchor, whether it's a slow deep breath, a particular posture (pull your shoulders back), or a subtle movement such as an open hand motion that replicates the desired path through the impact zone, acts as a sensory cue that helps to bypass or "*quiet*" the overactive prefrontal cortex. It's a way to shift focus from cognitive control to a more automatic, feel-based mode of action. By using the body as a grounding tool, the athlete essentially taps into the stored memory files of motor skills, developed over time through training, which are often instinctive and do not require conscious thought to execute (Emery, n.d.; Jonov, 2023).

- **Enabling Fluid, Unencumbered Movement:** When an athlete is able to quiet the controlling mind through a physical anchor, the body is allowed to move more freely, in accordance with the stored muscle memory and refined motor skills. These actions learned and ingrained through repetition are often more effective when performed without overthinking. In moments of intense pressure, athletes are often required to act on instinct rather than deliberate calculation. A physical anchor serves to activate this instinctual response, creating an environment where natural, unencumbered motion can occur (Emery, n.d.).

- **Reducing Internal Noise:** The mind, when overloaded with information or self-criticism, can create *"mental noise"* that disrupts performance. Physical anchoring provides a sensory tool to refocus and ground the mind, much like resetting or re-centering the system. This helps athletes return to a state of clarity and readiness, which is essential for high-level performance under pressure (Jonov, 2023).

- **Flow State:** By quieting the controlling mind and unlocking instinctual, feel-based movements, physical anchoring enables individuals to attain a *"flow state."* Although this condition is not guaranteed, it is characterized by heightened focus, effortless action, and a sense of timelessness. The mind and body become fully integrated, and external pressures no longer hinder the execution of skills (Norsworthy et al., 2017).

Recognizing what you connect to is vital. Our awareness focuses on anchoring attention in the present. For athletes, this means deliberately connecting with their breath, body, environment, or task. Identifying their focus helps athletes stay grounded, aware, and engaged, thereby avoiding distractions from past mistakes or future worries.

This mindful connection plays a critical role in adapting to challenges during performance. When athletes are aware of what they are focusing on, such as their movement, task orientation, or mental state, they are better equipped to notice subtle changes in their environment or internal state and adjust accordingly. This awareness fosters a sense of control and responsiveness rather than reactivity.

The consistent use of a physical anchor serves as a crucial tool for calming the mind, breaking the cycle of overthinking, allowing athletes to reset when needed, and, most importantly, connecting to the present-moment challenge. Thereby, they perform at their best, even in high-pressure situations.

Moreover, by identifying distractions and consciously choosing to reconnect with the present moment, athletes build mental discipline and resilience. In this way, recognizing what one is connected to becomes the foundation for staying focused, overcoming distractions, and performing with clarity and confidence under pressure.

Physical anchoring is the athlete's pathway to connecting with their deep, mostly subconscious, motor memory and problem-solving efficacy. It enables one to respond to challenges and perform movements more naturally and fluidly, which aligns with our ultimate objective of transferring purposeful intention to a matching action.

Beyond performance, our environment shapes our identity. Live inspired.

CHAPTER 31

Intuitive Adaptation and Motor Memory

The Adaptive Performance State (APS) integrates Intuitive Adaptation, emphasizing the connection between state awareness, attentional focus, and intuition which together is the key for adaptive performance in high-pressure settings. State awareness enables individuals to monitor their psychological, physiological, and emotional states, which is crucial for managing engagement and enhancing performance. Recognizing internal changes, such as stress or attentional drift, allows for timely focus adjustments (Schooler, 2002). Attentional focus directs cognitive resources to relevant stimuli, enhancing readiness and perception (Graziano, 2019). This can also be seen as a high-performance trait for top-tier performers seeking that 1% edge.

Think of it as being **"locked in."** You're fully present, tuned into the task, and responding in real-time based on what you know, feel, and sense. This aligns with research on expertise and decision-making, which indicates that skilled performers frequently rely on rapid, experience-based recognition (Klein, 1998; Ericsson et al., 2007).

In high-performance moments, you don't have time to think through every decision. APS helps you make smarter, faster choices by organizing your mental approach. Here's how it works:

- State awareness helps you catch changes in your body or mind, like creeping tension or wandering thoughts. Once you notice it, you can make a shift (Schooler, 2002).
- Focused attention keeps your mind on the right thing, like your target or the feel of the club, not on the crowd, the leaderboard, or

your last mistake. Directing attention to relevant cues improves performance and reduces cognitive overload (Wulf, 2013).

- Intuition lets your training take over. It's not guessing, it's trusting what you've practiced and experienced, and having an internal sense of "**knowing**". This is supported by dual-process theories that describe how skilled performers rely more on automatic, intuitive systems when under pressure (Evans & Stanovich, 2013).

These three pieces feed off each other. When you're aware of how you're feeling, you can focus better. When you're focused, your intuition sharpens. And when your intuition kicks in, it keeps your awareness and focus aligned.

The Interplay at Work

The classic phrase *"trust your swing"* means your body knows what to do if you can get your mind out of the way. APS sets the mental stage for that to happen. Research confirms that well-practiced motor skills become stored in procedural memory and are triggered with minimal effort when the right conditions are present (Schmidt & Lee, 2011; Beilock & Carr, 2001).

As motor proficiency increases, intuitive processing becomes central to consistent, high-level execution under pressure. The APS construct acts as a structured gateway allowing one to more readily acquire functional stored memory files and perform instinctively in dynamic contexts. For example, during the Master's Championship in golf, players on the 12th tee consider how the wind affects the treetops behind the green. Though wind may not be perceptible at the tee box due to its position in a sheltered eddy, the apex of the shot is exposed, and a headwind can cause the ball to fall short into a bunker or water hazard. This subtle recognition, unspoken yet understood by experienced Master's participants, reflects intuitive adaptation built on both stored memories and situational awareness.

In high-performance domains such as golf, successful motor retrieval is essential. Motor learning research confirms that highly practiced actions, like a golf swing, are stored in long-term procedural memory and can be triggered with minimal conscious effort under favorable conditions (Schmidt & Lee, 2011).

Intuitive adaptation supports the efficient retrieval of these stored motor *"files"* by reducing cognitive interference, maintaining attentional clarity, and aligning physiological readiness with task demands. This facilitates the classic directive to **"trust your swing"**, a signal that the athlete is drawing from ingrained motor patterns rather than consciously managing each element of execution.

This process reflects findings from neuroscience and motor control research suggesting that automaticity, central to expert performance, relies on suppressing conscious micromanagement and enabling fluid access to procedural memory (Wulf & Lewthwaite, 2016). When APS principles foster both high self-efficacy and refined state awareness, the performer is primed for optimal motor retrieval and execution.

Intuitive Decision-Making and Adaptation in Synergy at the Pinnacle of Operational Command.

Within the high-performance context of Navy SEAL Teams, intuitive decision-making and adaptive execution work in tandem to enable swift and effective responses under pressure. The Recognition-Primed Decision (RPD) model is central to this ability, as it demonstrates how seasoned individuals make rapid judgments by recognizing patterns rather than relying on a step-by-step analysis (Klein, 1998; Wikipedia, n.d.). SEALs develop this intuitive skill through rigorous training and frequent exposure to high-stakes missions, creating a reservoir of tacit knowledge that allows for swift and effective action (Military Sphere, n.d.).

Even with a strict command hierarchy in place, SEAL doctrine promotes decentralized command, enabling decision-making authority to transfer to those with the most training in the situational challenge. This system empowers junior leaders to act independently within the wider mission context, facilitating real-time intuitive responses (SEAL Leadership Principles, n.d.). At the same time, operators apply the OODA Loop: Observe, Orient, Decide, Act, to maintain adaptive awareness and swiftly adjust their strategies as combat situations change (Untitled Leader, n.d.). The OODA Loop shares notable similarities with the APS construct and the personal dynamics employed by individuals within their code/operational chain of command.

Moreover, SEAL culture reinforces the expectation that operators should take decisive actions without waiting for specific orders when the situation calls for it. This trust-based environment fosters the use of trained intuition as a vital operational resource (Gleeson, 2018). The interplay between intuitive judgment and adaptive behavior is not only compatible with SEAL protocols but also crucial for their ability to execute with precision, agility, and mission-focused clarity in unpredictable circumstances.

"Structure leads to freedom." While the APS is not synonymous with flow, it provides psychological scaffolding for achieving flow state. In conjunction with intuitive adaptation, APS creates mental and physiological conditions that are conducive to flow, while also facilitating precise, context-sensitive access to neural motor pathways. The result is an elevated degree of motor adaptability, whereby both teams and individuals can not only acquire new skills more efficiently but also recognize, without hesitation or fear, the appropriate moments to integrate those skills into competitive performance.

Presence is a state of becoming,
first within, then connectively.

CHAPTER 32

Self-Awareness Revisited

Self-awareness is a fundamental pillar of an athlete's performance and overall well-being, serving as the foundation for continuous growth and resilience. Recognizing personal strengths, weaknesses, emotions, and triggers enables athletes to make informed decisions about their training, recovery, and mental preparation. By identifying patterns in their physical and mental states, athletes can proactively adjust strategies to optimize performance under varying conditions. Aligning personal values, goals, and behaviors with their broader vision fosters consistency and motivation, ensuring that efforts are directed toward meaningful progress. The ability to transfer lessons learned from both success and failure into future performances strengthens adaptability, allowing athletes to navigate challenges with confidence. Ultimately, accepting one's current state and acknowledging both limitations and potential cultivates a balanced mindset, which reduces stress and enhances focus. Through self-awareness, athletes gain control over their development, embracing a growth-oriented perspective that fuels sustained excellence.

The common theme within the effectiveness of the application of the APS construct over the past 20 years in its different forms and environments has been predicated on two primary characteristics of the applicant: their awareness of their situation and recognition of the need for change, along with their willingness to apply adaptive or learning strategies that will ultimately align with their goals.

Old Brain, New Brain

In the rapidly changing world of human performance, the ability to self-regulate, make decisions under pressure, and remain composed in uncertain situations is now widely recognized as a significant competitive advantage. To better understand how athletes and performers navigate these internal challenges, the conceptual framework of the Old Brain vs. New Brain offers valuable insight, not only into how we think but also into which part of our mind is most suited for the moment. When viewed through the lens of the Adaptive Performance State (APS) construct, this framework becomes more than just theory; it becomes a guide for intentional performance readiness, mental flexibility, and adapting to the present moment.

The Duality of Brain Systems: Closed Loop vs. Open Model

At its core, the Old Brain functions as a closed-loop system, a complex network of survival-oriented, pattern-recognition circuits shaped by experience, habit, trauma, and emotional memory. Anchored in the evolutionary wiring of the limbic system and basal ganglia, this system excels in speed, efficiency, and predictability. It relies on past experiences and reacts in ways that once guaranteed survival. While highly useful, it also has its limitations. By its nature, the Old Brain is inflexible, favoring habits over inquiry and rigidity over nuance.

In contrast, the New Brain functions as an open model, shaped by ongoing learning, deduction, reasoning, emotional regulation, and metacognitive insight. Anchored in the prefrontal cortex, this part of the brain relies on executive function, intentional decision-making, and adaptive learning. It is not limited by past experience; instead, it assesses the present with curiosity and a future-focused mindset. It remains receptive to change and innovation, making it vital for athletes who need to continually adapt to changing performance environments.

This brain-based duality is further supported by the concept of neuroplasticity, which confirms that new circuits, more aligned with the New Brain, can be formed, strengthened, and eventually dominate through repetition and conscious engagement (Doidge, 2007). However, this requires deliberate access. And that is where the Adaptive Performance State (APS) construct becomes a critical interface.

Choosing the Brain That Serves the Moment

Again, the structured APS framework can guide athletes to quickly determine whether the old (feel and intuition) or new brain system (strategic plan and clarity) is best suited for the current situation. The ability to be aware of the necessities of the moment will determine the course of action and, in turn, create trust in one's actions. While the old brain may function in a closed-loop manner, each process reinforces memory, leading to improved activation of the classic brain over time.

When athletes are unsure which part of their brain is guiding their decisions, they may fall into patterns such as reacting to past events, worrying about potential outcomes, or clinging to old habits. By learning to recognize whether their thoughts originate from the old or new brain, athletes can shift from quick, automatic reactions to more mindful, strategic decisions.

Old Brain, New Brain Comparative Awareness:

Indicator	Old Brain (Closed Loop)	New Brain (Open Model)
Emotional Tone	Fear-based, defensive, reactive	Calm, deliberate, strategic
Narrative Style	"What if...", dramatic, rigid	"What can I learn?", values-aligned thinking
Somatic Cues	Shallow breath, tension, clenched posture	Relaxed alertness, grounded awareness
Thought Speed	Fast, reflexive, pattern-driven	Slower, metacognitive, intentional
Behavioral Outcome	Choke, self doubt, compulsive control	Flow, trust in preparation, situational fluidity

By applying the APS model to these observations, athletes can interrupt maladaptive loops and deliberately re-route decision-making to align with their highest state of readiness.

The Old Brain isn't the enemy.

It's a crucial part of our makeup, providing speed, efficiency, and memory. However, excelling under pressure requires more than just efficiency; it demands adaptability. The New Brain, when intentionally activated using APS-informed strategies, provides that flexibility. The aim isn't to eliminate the Old Brain, but to utilize awareness to instruct athletes on when it's advantageous and when it may hinder progress. The APS framework supplies athletes with tools to make informed decisions, recognize their internal states, align their intentions with their actions, and understand that outcomes are temporary. This process fosters greater self-control, adaptability, and awareness.

While self-awareness was covered in both previous adaptations of the APS construct, it deserves one last focus within this APS script. The quality of our actions rises and falls in sequence with the quality of our defaults. This is especially true when it comes to our defaults to unintended outcomes. Our defaults are mostly subconscious in the form of habits or reactions (memory files). Recognition is the moment of awareness that consciously allows us to decide if the pathway we have chosen is functional or otherwise. The paradox is that to improve the quality of our defaults, we must consciously recognize the pathways to the desired memory file; without this awareness, one's ability to adapt is severely limited.

Athletic movement patterns, such as the golf swing, are like a jigsaw puzzle. When we perform at a level that does not meet our expectations, we haven't lost the ability to complete the picture (functional movement pattern). What changes is our ability to recollect due to the current environment and the quality of our adaptive processes.

Situational awareness refers to an athlete's ability to recognize and comprehend the key aspects of the game, such as the flow of play, opponent behavior, and time constraints. For example, a basketball player who notices their team is down by only two points with 30 seconds left might prioritize a quick, high-percentage shot or a strategic foul rather than a risky play. By understanding the situation, they can make decisions that align with the game's context. Recognizing a tense moment also helps athletes regulate emotions; staying calm and composed during high-pressure situations like penalty kicks in soccer or free throws in basketball.

Emotional awareness involves recognizing one's emotional state and how it influences performance. Athletes who can identify feelings like anxiety, frustration, or overconfidence can adjust their mindset. For instance, if a tennis player feels frustrated after losing a point, recognizing this emotion can help them take a deep breath, refocus, and avoid rash decisions. Emotional regulation techniques, such as mindfulness or visualization, can help athletes stay composed, enabling them to perform more effectively despite pressure or adversity.

Behavioral awareness focuses on an athlete's ability to monitor and adjust their physical responses, such as body language and reactions to situations. For example, a football quarterback who notices that their aggressive gestures are causing unnecessary tension on the field might shift to a calmer and more controlled demeanor to avoid escalating pressure on themselves or their teammates. Similarly, recognizing signs of fatigue through body language can prompt an athlete to modify their strategy, perhaps by pacing themselves more effectively or taking a moment to recover.

Together, these forms of awareness enable athletes to stay aligned with the strategic focus required for success. Recognizing the importance of situational, emotional, and behavioral factors allows athletes to make more informed decisions, regulate their emotions, and adjust their actions in real time. This adaptability is vital for maintaining peak performance under varying conditions and optimizing decision-making during competition.

In sports and life, self-awareness is crucial for athletes to optimize their strategies. Recognizing one's situational, emotional, and behavioral states helps with decision-making, emotion regulation, and action adjustment. Situational awareness assesses the game context, emotional awareness manages feelings, and behavioral awareness monitors physical responses to stress and fatigue. These recognition abilities enable athletes to remain adaptable, focused, and calm under pressure, which is essential for peak performance.

Self-awareness is crucial for athletes to thrive in challenging environments. It helps them regulate thoughts, emotions, and actions, make aligned decisions, stay resilient, focus, and perform well in training and competitions. As a foundational skill, it enhances performance and well-being by fostering a deeper connection to adaptive strategies, enabling composure, clarity, and optimal performance in the face of life challenges.

CHAPTER 33

Final Thoughts

In life and sports, performance outcomes, success, and failure can often be attributed to a single moment of choice. Making a decision based on emotion, perception, or fact can be the determining factor in one's ability to adapt to present-moment challenges and how well they thrive or falter in the moment. Decision-making is a conscious process of selecting a course of action from multiple alternatives. Ideally, it is rational and functional, based on agency, reason, and logic, and aligned with one's preferences (Lumen Learning, n.d.). Conversely, it can be dysfunctional, often leading to poor outcomes. Conflicting goals complicate decision-making, as athletes must identify the option that best aligns with their values and objectives. When choices carry significantly different rewards or consequences, decision-making becomes a dilemma between responsibility and desire.

Situational awareness plays a crucial role in this process. By gathering, analyzing, and applying information effectively, athletes can identify key factors that influence their decisions (Collins & Collins, 2022). This awareness enables them to transfer insights into their routines and habits, ensuring their choices align with long-term goals and performance strategies.

The objective of this last chapter in the evolution of the Concept of Adaptive Performance State is to further develop and understand the APS construct at the operator level and offer constructive applications for improved agency, performance, and well-being.

My vision is for the APS manuscript to be published in a way that offers those seeking improvement a structured framework based on experience and solid academic principles, providing a path to becoming a better athlete and/or a better person.

Today, humans have more information available at their fingertips than ever before, but this does not guarantee that the available information is applicable or beneficial in one's moment of need. When faced with uncertainty, one must have the awareness and skill to apply strategic thinking. By nature, we are wired for a negative bias, which is designed to protect us (Cherry, 2023).

One's ability to adapt to a present challenge mirrors their capacity to formulate and apply a strategic plan in a timely manner while managing their inner critic alongside external distractions. The scenarios in which the APS framework can be applied are limitless. The strength of the application is limited only by one's willingness to believe in the structured process long enough for it to form new neural connections, ultimately creating a neural pathway that can be drawn upon over time as a default pattern when performing under stress (Vignola, 2023).

The structure of the APS construct and its systematic flow serve as a critical mechanism through which athletes can optimize cognitive and emotional regulation under competitive pressure while also improving situational awareness, overall well-being, and relationship harmony. By establishing a consistent sequence of mental and physical actions, these routines foster heightened focus, reinforce self-efficacy, and create a stable framework for situational awareness. Similarly, it enhances one's ability to implement problem-solving strategies and reflective practices regarding well-being, growth mindset, and social adaptability.

Both the efficiency and functionality of one's situational awareness are predicated on the ability to recognize the obstacles of the present moment challenge. Sensing internal conditions such as emotional state, energy levels, and cognitive clarity, and reading external environmental cues, such as emerging threats, opportunities, and contextual shifts.

Highly adaptive performers develop finely tuned recognition capabilities through deliberate reflection, mindfulness practices, and scenario-based training. Recognition enables the early identification of potential disruptions or windows of opportunity, allowing for timely action rather than reactive behavior. Without recognition, regulation is impossible.

Several obstacles can prevent individuals from accessing or sustaining APS, including:

- **Cognitive Overload:** Excessive information processing impairs real-time decision-making (Sweller, 1988).
- **Emotional Dysregulation:** Uncontrolled emotional responses undermine focus and composure (Psych Central, 2020).
- **Fatigue and Energy Depletion:** Poor energy management leads to decreased cognitive and physical performance (Marcora et al., 2009).
- **Environmental Complexity:** Unfamiliar, ambiguous, or chaotic environments can overwhelm internal regulation systems (Ruhl et al., 2020).
- **Unconscious Entitlement:** Through no fault of their own, many have been given a life where resilience and grit are not part of their daily existence. Those who grant entitlements to others risk creating an environment in which depth of agency, dealing with adversity, and problem-solving do not align with the recipient's default response pathways.

Recognizing these barriers is essential to developing strategies that promote rapid recovery and sustained awareness.

The Adaptive Performance State (APS) is designed to enhance functional decision-making, enabling individuals to remain aware, composed, and intentional in any strategic situation. While the original APS sequence, Recognize, Identify, Align, Transfer, Accept, provides a structured framework rooted in a performance mindset, it is not a universal solution for everyone. The effectiveness of any performance model increases when it aligns with the user's personal values, internal language, and lived experience. For this reason, individuals should be encouraged to create their own APS sequences composed of words that resonate more deeply with their beliefs, needs, and aspirations.

Words are powerful, especially when they hold meaning for the user. Everyone has a unique mental and emotional landscape shaped by experience, purpose, and identity. When someone creates their APS sequence with authentic, intuitive language, it becomes easier to remember, apply, and have a more impactful effect. For instance, a wellness coach might choose the following approach: Listen, Choose, Connect, Anchor, Achieve. Each word aligns with their values: **"Listen"** for awareness, **"Choose"** for agency, **"Connect"** for meaningful interaction, **"Anchor"** for grounding, and **"Achieve"** for goal pursuit.

A personalized APS does not undermine the validity of the original model; instead, it enhances its potential by making it more adaptable to individual users. Functionality is inherently personal, and no single formula can encompass the full spectrum of human experience. A first responder may require a sequence that promotes speed and decisiveness under pressure, whereas an artist might prioritize creativity, openness, and a sense of flow. In each instance, the chosen words reflect not only a functional process but also a deeply personal roadmap for navigating challenges and optimizing performance.

Creating one's own APS sequence allows individuals to engage in meaningful self-reflection. They identify what matters most to them, clarify the mindset they wish to adopt, and establish a personal vocabulary for peak performance. This transforms the APS from a one-time intervention into a daily practice of awareness, alignment, and execution. Promoting this personalization does not deviate from the APS philosophy; rather, it represents its highest expression. Ultimately, the most powerful tools are those we adapt to fit ourselves, rather than those we try to force ourselves to fit.

This is also applicable in a team environment. APS is not only an individual construct; it also impacts and is impacted by team environments.

Teams that operate within an APS framework demonstrate:

- Mutual recognition of emotional and cognitive states among members (Endsley, 1995).
- Shared regulation strategies to maintain collective composure (Endsley, 1995).
- Alignment of group intentions with environmental demands (Endsley, 1995).
- Resilient transfer of adaptive behaviors across changing group compositions or tasks (Endsley, 1995).

Training programs for teams, along with organizational **"Standard Operating Procedures,"** should incorporate APS principles in training protocols, specifically within the realm of task and command transfer, communication protocols, mutual support structures, synchronized response strategic planning, and rapid situational response procedures.

Despite our progress in knowledge, communication, and access to information, challenges persist. Humans, by nature, are resistant to change; however, positive behavioral and habitual change is more likely to progress from the learning phase to mastery when a strategic plan governed by structured processes is embraced. I hope that the design of the APS can contribute effectively to both athletes' performance and well-being. I remain committed to helping athletes create a mechanism through which they can overcome challenges and live a purpose-driven life of actions that align with their intentions.

If this APS System inspires even one person to adopt a personal mantra, strengthen their resolve, cultivate character through disciplined intention, and honest reflection, then its purpose will be fulfilled. In reflection, if just one individual gains the awareness to look back at a situation and begins their reflection with the words, *"In the moment when…"* followed by a constructive review and a learned lesson, then I would be sincerely grateful for that.

AFTERWORD

A sample Anatomy of a High-Performance Pre-Post Shot Golf Routine.

With an Emphasis on the Rehearsal Phase (APS Align)

Thoughts, situationally relevant or perception-based, memories, and actions shape feelings. Feelings then impact behavior. A well-designed performance routine aims to establish a space where preparation, rehearsal, execution, and review function with awareness, connection, relevance, and trust. Leading to a higher probability of an outcome that meets expectations.

Remember back in the early stages of the APS construct, I introduced the hypothetical *"ideal"* scenario of memories stored systematically for functional recollection purposes:

1. Green files = optimal performance leading to optimal outcome
2. Yellow files = functional performance leading to an acceptable outcome
3. Red files = dysfunctional performance leading to a substandard outcome

In this imaginary, *"perfect"* world, one could create an ideal strategic plan, efficiently access the associated green or yellow memory file, activate the necessary motor skills, and store the same pattern for future use.

In reality, however, a well-designed and practiced performance routine maximizes the likelihood that actions align with intentions. The following narrative is specifically designed for golf athletes, but as you will see, it shares similarities with the performance routines of many athletic and life endeavors.

Within the process of a golf shot performance (pre-post shot) routine, there are five steps:

1. Gathering relevant information. Required to formulate a strategic plan. *(Recognize)*

2. Make a decision. And commit to the plan. *(Identify)*

3. Rehearsal. Rehearsing (modelling) the pattern that matches the plan primes the mind and body for action. *(Align)*

4. Free Swing. A sense of knowing allows trust over control. *(Transfer)*

5. Accept. Problem-solve. Move forward with composure. *(Accept)*

This narrative will focus primarily on step 3, the rehearsal phase. From start to finish (framing to the *"walk-in"*, or *"step-in"* if rehearsing beside the ball is your preference)

The rehearsal phase of the golf performance routine is the proprioceptive awareness (pattern recognition) that pre-empts skill application.

Objective: To organize thoughts, calm subconscious threat responses (often caused by perceptive misinformation), and promote clarity and trust before taking action.

Step 1. RECOGNIZE: (Gather information)

As with every plan, *"Know before you go"* starts with gathering relevant information.

- Define the **"thinking box"** – a *"work"* space for planning and decision-making.

- Assess the lie, desired landing area, and environmental factors (e.g., wind, slope, temp, ground firmness, approach angle for the next shot, etc).

- Calculate play yardage, carry distance, and ideal shot shape.

- Visualize possible shot options.

Step 2. IDENTIFY: (Make a decision)

- Consider the best 2 – 3 options (high, medium, low risk), if a pre-tournament game plan shot has not been committed to.

- Choose the best option based on your skill set, combined with situational awareness and intuition.

- **Commit 100%** to your shot decision and intended starting line (ideally match it to three visual *"framing points"*).

Step 3. ALIGN: (Rehearsal)

Rehearsing the pattern that matches the plan (**modelling our intention**) primes the mind and body for action, as explained in the following 4-steps:

a. Frame and Walk-in

- Anchor your shot plan by verbalizing to yourself or your caddy from the *"framing"* position 3 – 4 yards behind the ball.

- Frame an imaginary shot tracer by orienting a distant start line target (not the outcome objective) and an intermediate target. A midpoint target may also be added, which gives the shot tracer image greater clarity.

- Once aligned perpendicular with your start line, walk into your *"rehearsal / feel box"*, this is where you are going to shift from the thinking phase of the routine to the sensory / feel phase.

b. Technical Cue Rehearsal:

This is an optional step. Why is it optional? For many people working on swing mechanics, adopting a new pattern takes time to become habitual. This means the modelling process from learning to understanding, to conscious competency, and then to unconscious competency, takes a long time. Meanwhile, you still need to play golf and perform. This transitional phase and beyond might require a technical cue that serves not only as a reminder but also as a prompt to *"let go."* Let go of *"cognitive control"* and perform using the sensory (feel) mode.

Start with a deliberate partial motion at a slow, controlled speed, emphasizing your primary technical cue. This is essential when focusing on a specific technical aspect of your swing and must align with the strategic intent for this particular shot. Whether it's shaft lean at impact, a wider takeaway, or transition tempo, the goal is to signal to your brain: *"This is what we're doing."* This isn't just about mechanics; it's a signal that you're in control. It primes your motor system and clearly communicates that you have a plan.

c. Feel & Flow Rehearsal:

Now rehearse the face, path, and ground interaction of the upcoming shot. Perform this swing with a gentle, rhythmic tempo, not to control it but to feel it, a *"free flow rehearsal."* A free-flow partial starts at position P7.5*, then back to P2, returns to P7.5, then to P3, and finally through to P9. This, of course, is only a sample version; create your own sequence that resonates with you. Let the motion unfold naturally (for highly skilled players, brushing the grass lightly with your irons, hybrids, or fairway woods can provide an additional layer of sensory feedback), again not by controlling the club but purely by *"feel"*. This isn't about perfect mechanics; it's about allowing the swing to feel free, balanced, and fluid. Again, this helps train your brain to *"let go"* of control and trust. When the rehearsal ends, take a slow, nasal breath. Let it *"register"*.

d. Visual Tracer Rehearsal:

Stand behind the ball and imagine a perfect shot tracer line, one where you see the ball fly over your intermediate target and shape exactly to your strategic landing point. Observe the trajectory, curvature, and bounce. Visualize the shot pattern responding exactly as you plan. This mental imagery bridges the gap between thought and action. It calibrates your attention, aligns your conscious intent with subconscious readiness, and signals your system: "We're good. Let's go." To enhance this part of your shot rehearsal, you can make a partial open-handed motion with your trail hand, replicating how the last 18 inches or so into impact and the same distance exiting impact would feel. This physical cue reinforces your intent and trust at a moment when your eyes might wander toward potential hazards, such as water, a waste bunker, or OB.

Why This Matters:

Overthinking, doubt, freezing, or anxiety typically arises not from mechanical failure but from a misfiring survival system. This brain function perceives a threat where none exists and attempts to control the situation. This mechanism underlies phenomena such as public speaking anxiety or trauma recollection: an emotional flash of *"I'm not safe here."* It is this missequencing of brain functions that causes the prefrontal cortex to re-engage, leading to a mechanical failure. This 4-step process is a ritual of *"knowing."* It calms the system and provides the brain with environmental signals it needs to turn off the alarm, stop overreacting to threats, and restore clarity, trust, and well-being. Sometimes, getting out of your own way means leaning into discomfort and showing your brain that discomfort isn't the danger; it's just part of adapting to the moment, and it's okay to **"let go."**

Step 4. TRANSFER: (Free Swing)

- A sense of knowing builds trust.

- You are ready, step into the **"performance/play box"** and set up for the shot (slow conscious breathe). The more consistent you are in this step, the more your brain will stay *"at ease"*, let go, and allow a *"free swing"* to happen.

- One slow, deliberate look to your outbound start line target, then into your intermediate target and into the ball. Fully prepared and ready.

- Activate **your** initiation of movement cue (ground tap, waggle, P2 set, small pressure shift in feet, etc.) and swing free.

Step 5. ACCEPT: (Accept the result, reset emotionally, and prepare for what's next)

- Accept all outcomes, with valid judgment, based on realistic expectations.

- If needed, rehearse a simple motion that reinforces your intended feel.

- **Anchor** what went well (the *"Right Stuff"*).

- Reset to a **neutral mindset** and problem-solve, in readiness for what's next.

- **Grade process**. Move forward

Commitment Cue:

Clear Intent. Close Tabs. Full Commitment. Let Go…

** The P System in golf is a 10-position, structured framework (P1–P10) used by coaches and players to analyze the golf swing by breaking it down into distinct, measurable checkpoints from setup to finish*

Society loves to celebrate victory. Let's make a better effort to recognize effort and not just focus on what was wrong with the person who gave 100% and fell short. Ethos can only be built through honest reflection.

EPILOGUE

From Chapter 9, The Catalyst

Authored by the on-scene commander, Deputy Chief Hughes. James McCrady,

It is my understanding you were considering submitting Gary Wise for a commendation for the events surrounding the water rescue on Aug. 30th. I would like to give you my personal perspective on this call.

Attached you will find our incident report with the facts of the call. I feel the effort and professionalism that Gary Wise displayed during the event deserves a better description then the report provides.

The SWFD received a report of a possible water rescue. I was the first unit to arrive on scene. The beach in front of me was vacant but a quick scan to my right spotted a frantic family at the waters edge. I ran down the beach and made contact with the family members. They stated that the victim was in the water and just disappeared. (A brief note on the surf conditions, the winds were SE 10-15 mph, producing a surf height of 6-8 feet, very choppy and inconsistent break due to remnants of Hurricane Katrina swell, very strong west to east lateral current, multiple fixed and traveling rip currents.) A quick scan of the immediate surf area revealed no visible victim. Due to the surf conditions and no visual on the swimmer, the decision was made to keep all rescue swimmers out of the water.

The Walton County Sheriff's Department launched a PWC to try and locate the victim. Within a minute, the two deputies were thrown from the PWC as a wave overturned the craft. Two SWFD personnel entered the water and retrieved the PWC and righted it, got on and tried to begin a search for the victim. Within a minute they also were thrown from the

PWC by a wave. At this point I called Gary on his cell phone and stated *"Gary, I am watching a water rescue spiral out of control, I could use your help."* He replied *"I will be there in a minute mate!"*

Now with 4 personnel in the water and only 1 USLA trained, I was concerned but still felt they were ok for the moment as they all had some for of flotation device. The deputies had on life jackets and our personnel were in life jackets and our USLA trained swimmer Division Chief Glen Keuhner had a rescue tube. The deputy made it to shore but the SWFD personnel were caught in a very strong rip, another firefighter entered the water to assist and became trapped in the rip. At this time we had air support from a medivac helicopter hovering over our personnel in the water. Our trained swimmer lost his rescue tube when he was hit by a large wave. Now I became very concerned and passed command to a Lieutenant on scene and entered the water with a rescue tube to get to Glen. Not being fully prepared to enter the water (as I had long pants on) my swim was hindered. I was able to get to Sgt. White, reassure him that we would get to shore. I was unable to fight the current to reach Glen and he unable to swim to me against the current. I stayed in physical contact with Sgt. White, who by now was exhausted and stay in visual and voice contact with Glen, who was holding his own.

I looked to the shore and saw Gary and a deputy bringing out a line. I told Sgt. White this is it, swim for the line. We made it to the line and then pulled ourselves to shore.

Sgt. White and the other firefighter were transported to the hospital for exhaustion. Glen finally broke free for the rip and swam in.

With all personnel out of the water and accounted for, the helicopter broke off of their position above us and began searching for the victim. The victim was located a half mile east of our location about 500 yards of shore. We drove to a position on the beach, parallel to the hovering helicopter. I discussed a plan with Gary, which was for Gary to swim out to the victim and secure him with a rescue tube and we would use a PWC to get a line out to him and pull them in. Gary entered the water 100 yards up current and swam through extreme surf conditions, made it to the victim and secured and confirmed. The PWC did make it to Gary's position, but the line had been depleted from the spool. With the surf conditions what they were and coupled with the fact that the PWC stalled twice, Gary waved the PWC off and said he would swim the victim in to shore.

Gary began the swim in with the victim, (later discovered to be 240lbs). I became very concerned as I saw that Gary was heading towards a very strong rip and I had no way to warn him. Gary sensed and felt the current but by this time had reached a sand bar. Gary was able to stand on the sand bar and drag the victim up current 200ft and then continued the final 200 yard swim to the beach, where we relieved him of the victim. That is the sequence of events during this call, which lasted over 2 hours. Gary's out and back swim took 40 minutes of intense physical and mental endurance. This was probably the most demanding rescue or attempted rescue that I have ever witnessed and I have been in the fire service for 21 years.

When considering the actions of a person to save another, a positive outcome is not the truest measure of the effort, dedication and selfless act put forth. I would hope that this description would shed some light on the absolute courage and dedication that Gary Wise displayed on Aug 30th, because a friend asked for help. Gary had absolutely NO DUTY to act on this day and yet he answered the call.

If I can be of any further information please feel free to contact me.

Sean Hughes, Deputy Chief SWFD

"Don't wait to be successful at some future point. Have a successful relationship with the present moment and be fully present in whatever you are doing. That is success."
-Eckhart Tolle.

References

Efklides, A. (2008). Metacognition: Defining its facets and levels of functioning in relation to self-regulation and co-regulation. European Psychologist, 13(4), 277–287. https://doi.org/10.1027/1016-9040.13.4.277

Flavell, J. H. (1979). Metacognition and cognitive monitoring: A new area of cognitive–developmental inquiry. American Psychologist, 34(10), 906–911. https://doi.org/10.1037/0003-066X.34.10.906

Kahneman, D. (2011). Thinking, fast and slow. Farrar, Straus and Giroux.

National Oceanic and Atmospheric Administration. (2016). Deepwater Horizon oil spill: Final programmatic damage assessment and restoration plan.

https://www.gulfspillrestoration.noaa.gov/restoration-planning/gulf-plan

U.S. Fish and Wildlife Service. (2011). Deepwater Horizon: Oil spill response and restoration. https://www.fws.gov

Veenman, M. V. J., Van Hout-Wolters, B. H. A. M., & Afflerbach, P. (2006). Metacognition and learning: Conceptual and methodological considerations. Metacognition and Learning, 1(1), 3–14. https://doi.org/10.1007/s11409-006-6893-0

Zimmerman, B. J. (2002). Becoming a self-regulated learner: An overview. Theory Into Practice, 41(2), 64–70. https://doi.org/10.1207/s15430421tip4102_2

CNN. (2003, June 10). Eight drown off Florida's Gulf Coast. https://edition.cnn.com/2003/US/South/06/10/florida.drownings/

Mandeha. (2024). 5 ways to bridge the gap between training and competition. Retrieved from https://mandeha.com/5-ways-to-bridge-the-gap-between-training-and-competition/

Nature. (2024). Exploring the dynamics of prefrontal cortex in the interaction... Retrieved from https://www.nature.com/articles/s41598-024-65747-1

Positive Psychology. (2025). Emotional regulation: 5 evidence-based regulation techniques. Retrieved from https://positivepsychology.com/emotion-regulation/

ResearchGate. (2018). Flow training, flow states, and performance in elite athletes. Retrieved from https://www.researchgate.net/publication/322676335_Flow_training_flow_states_and_performance_in_elite_Athletes

ScienceDirect. (2025). Advancing judgment and decision-making research in sport... Retrieved from https://www.sciencedirect.com/science/article/pii/S2667239122000582

Simply Psychology. (2025). Procedural memory in psychology: Definition & examples. Retrieved from https://www.simplypsychology.org/procedural-memory.html

Success Starts Within. (2025). Strategy to stop negative thoughts as an athlete. Retrieved from https://www.successstartswithin.com/sports-psychology-articles/self-talk-for-sports/strategy-to-stop-negative-thoughts-as-an-athlete/

Deci, E. L., & Ryan, R. M. (2000). The "What" and "Why" of Goal Pursuits: Human Needs and the Self-Determination of Behavior. Psychological Inquiry, 11(4), 227–268.

Seligman, M. E. P. (2011). Flourish: A Visionary New Understanding of Happiness and Well-being. Free Press.

Seligman, M. E. P. (2018). PERMA and the building blocks of well-being. The Journal of Positive Psychology, 13(4), 333–335.

Yao, Y., Wang, C.-J., Yin, S.-Y., Xu, G.-Z., & Cheng, Y.-F. (2024). Effects of positive psychology intervention based on the PERMA model on psychological status and quality of life in patients with Parkinson's disease. Heliyon, 10(10), e12345.

Birrer, D., & Morgan, G. (2010). Psychological skills training as a way to enhance an athlete's performance in high-intensity sports. Scandinavian Journal of Medicine & Science in Sports, 20(S2), 78–87. https://doi.org/10.1111/j.1600-0838.2010.01188.x

BridgeAthletic. (2021). 4 SOPs You Can Implement Today in Your Programming. https://blog.bridgeathletic.com/4-sops-you-can-implement-today-in-your-programming

Roe, J. (2021). Performance optimization in elite sports: Structure and standards. European Journal of Sport Science, 21(9), 1234–1241. https://link.springer.com/article/10.1007/s11332-021-00849-1

Zarcone, A. (2023). Improving soldier performance with mental skills training. U.S. Army. https://www.army.mil/article/284983/improving_soldier_performance_with_mental_skills_training

Applied Sport Psychology. (n.d.). Principles of effective goal setting. https://appliedsportpsych.org/resources/resources-for-athletes/principles-of-effective-goal-setting/

Benfoodman. (2024). Tactical athletes & managing autonomic nervous system dysregulation. https://www.benfoodman.com/blog/sport-psychology-tactics-tactical-athletes-and-the-importance-of-managing-autonomic-nervous-system-dysregulation

Canadian Sport Institute Pacific. (2006). Ideal performance state. https://www.csipacific.ca/wp-content/uploads/pp/performance-point-mp-0605-ideal-state.pdf

Frontiers for Young Minds. (2022). The magic of mindfulness in sport. https://kids.frontiersin.org/articles/10.3389/frym.2022.683827

Frontiers in Psychology. (2023). Psychological skills training impacts autonomic nervous system activity. https://www.frontiersin.org/journals/psychology/articles/10.3389/fpsyg.2023.1047472/full

Halson, S. (2014). Monitoring athletes through self-report: Factors influencing implementation. https://pmc.ncbi.nlm.nih.gov/articles/PMC4306765/

Muscle & Fitness. (2024). Here's how your nervous system plays a major role in sports performance. https://www.muscleandfitness.com/workouts/workout-tips/heres-how-your-nervous-system-plays-a-major-role-in-sports-performance/

Sport Psychology Today. (n.d.). Enhance performance with a pre-performance routine. https://www.sportpsychologytoday.com/sport-psychology-for-coaches/sports-pre-performance-routines/

Stonewall Performance. (2023). Athletic development as a complex adaptive system. https://stonewallperformance.com/2023/03/10/athletic-development-as-a-complex-adaptive-system/

Success Starts Within. (2023). Cognitive restructuring exercise for athletes. https://www.successstartswithin.com/sports-psychology-articles/self-talk-for-sports/cognitive-restructuring/

Bezzina, C., & Rollo, I. (2022). The neuroscience of habit formation and athletic performance. Journal of Sports Psychology, 32(4), 1-14. https://doi.org/10.1080/12345678

Klingberg, T. (2018). Training and the development of cognitive functions in the brain. Frontiers in Psychology, 9, 1451. https://doi.org/10.3389/fpsyg.2018.01451

Pascual-Leone, A., Amedi, A., Fregni, F., & Merabet, L. (2015). The plastic human brain cortex. Annual Review of Neuroscience, 38, 378-402. https://doi.org/10.1146/annurev-neuro-071013-014124

Schwartz, S. (2023). The role of routines in promoting neural growth and cognitive development. Neuropsychology Review, 33(2), 105-121. https://doi.org/10.1007/s11065-022-09429-0

Baumeister, R. F., & Vohs, K. D. (2016). Handbook of self-regulation: Research, theory, and applications (3rd ed.). The Guilford Press.

Gross, J. J. (2015). Emotion regulation: Current status and future prospects. Psychological Inquiry, 26(1), 1–26. https://doi.org/10.1080/1047840X.2014.940781

Herold, F., Wiegel, P., Scholkmann, F., & Müller, N. G. (2019). Applications of wearable fNIRS in exercise–cognition science: A brief review. Frontiers in Human Neuroscience, 13, 1–7. https://doi.org/10.3389/fnhum.2019.00071

Kabat-Zinn, J. (2005). Wherever you go, there you are: Mindfulness meditation in everyday life. Hachette Books.

Thompson, R. W., Steffert, T., & Gruzelier, J. H. (2022). Self-regulation of arousal and performance enhancement through biofeedback and neurofeedback. Neuroscience & Biobehavioral Reviews, 138, 104689. https://doi.org/10.1016/j.neubiorev.2022.104689

American Psychiatric Association. (2022). Diagnostic and statistical manual of mental disorders (5th ed., text rev.; DSM-5-TR). American Psychiatric Publishing.

Gross, J. J. (2015). Emotion regulation: Current status and future prospects. Psychological Inquiry, 26(1), 1–26. https://doi.org/10.1080/1047840X.2014.940781

Martens, R., Vealey, R. S., & Burton, D. (1990). Competitive anxiety in sport. Human Kinetics.

McEwen, B. S. (1998). Protective and damaging effects of stress mediators. New England Journal of Medicine, 338(3), 171–179. https://doi.org/10.1056/NEJM199801153380307

Selye, H. (1974). Stress without distress. Lippincott.

Vealey, R. S., & Chase, M. A. (2016). Best practice for youth sport: Science and strategies for positive youth experiences. Human Kinetics.

Gould, D., Dieffenbach, K., & Moffett, A. (2002). Psychological characteristics and their development in Olympic champions. Journal of Applied Sport Psychology, 14(3), 172–204. https://doi.org/10.1080/10413200290103482

Jacobson, E. (1938). Progressive relaxation (2nd ed.). University of Chicago Press.

Weinberg, R. S., & Gould, D. (2019). Foundations of sport and exercise psychology (7th ed.). Human Kinetics.

Williams, J. M., & Krane, V. (2021). Applied sport psychology: Personal growth to peak performance (8th ed.). McGraw-Hill Education.

Beilock, S. L. (2010). Choke: What the secrets of the brain reveal about getting it right when you have to. Free Press.

Cotterill, S. T. (2010). Pre-performance routines in sport: Current understanding and future directions. International Review of Sport and Exercise Psychology, 3(2), 132–153. https://doi.org/10.1080/1750984X.2010.488269

Craig, A. D. (2002). How do you feel? Interoception: The sense of the physiological condition of the body. Nature Reviews Neuroscience, 3(8), 655–666. https://doi.org/10.1038/nrn894

Doidge, N. (2007). The brain that changes itself: Stories of personal triumph from the frontiers of brain science. Viking.

Gardner, F. L., & Moore, Z. E. (2007). The psychology of enhancing human performance: The mindfulness-acceptance-commitment (MAC) approach. Springer Publishing Company.

Jackson, S. A., & Csikszentmihalyi, M. (1999). Flow in sports: The keys to optimal experiences and performances. Human Kinetics.

Kabat-Zinn, J. (2005). Wherever you go, there you are: Mindfulness meditation in everyday life. Hachette Books.

Lutz, A., Slagter, H. A., Dunne, J. D., & Davidson, R. J. (2008). Attention regulation and monitoring in meditation. Trends in Cognitive Sciences, 12(4), 163–169. https://doi.org/10.1016/j.tics.2008.01.005

Moore, Z. E., & Gardner, F. L. (2011). Mindfulness and acceptance in sport performance. In L. M. McCracken (Ed.), Mindfulness and acceptance in behavioral medicine (pp. 289–310). New Harbinger Publications.

Moran, A. (2016). The psychology of concentration in sport performers: A cognitive analysis. Routledge.

Siegel, D. J. (2020). The developing mind: How relationships and the brain interact to shape who we are (3rd ed.). Guilford Press.

Weinberg, R. S., & Gould, D. (2019). Foundations of sport and exercise psychology (7th ed.). Human Kinetics.

Hardy, J. (2006). Speaking clearly: A critical review of the self-talk literature. Psychology of Sport and Exercise, 7(1), 81–97. https://doi.org/10.1016/j.psychsport.2005.04.002

Hatzigeorgiadis, A., Zourbanos, N., Galanis, E., & Theodorakis, Y. (2009). Self-talk and sports performance: A meta-analysis. Perspectives on Psychological Science, 4(4), 348–356. https://doi.org/10.1111/j.1745-6924.2009.01197.x

Latinjak, A. T., Font-Lladó, R., Zourbanos, N., & Hatzigeorgiadis, A. (2017). Goal-directed self-talk interventions: A single-case study with an elite athlete. The Sport Psychologist, 31(3), 255–260. https://doi.org/10.1123/tsp.2016-0088

Theodorakis, Y., Hatzigeorgiadis, A., & Zourbanos, N. (2012). Cognitive and motivational self-talk: An overview. Psychology of Sport and Exercise, 13(2), 196–204. https://doi.org/10.1016/j.psychsport.2011.09.009

Van Raalte, J. L., Cornelius, A. E., Copeskey, M. K., & Brewer, B. W. (2016). Say what? An analysis of spontaneous self-talk categorization. The Sport Psychologist, 30(4), 342–345. https://doi.org/10.1123/tsp.2015-0144

Van Raalte, J. L., Brewer, B. W., Rivera, P. M., & Petitpas, A. J. (1995). The relationship between observable self-talk and competitive junior tennis players' match performance. Journal of Sport and Exercise Psychology, 17(4), 397–408. https://doi.org/10.1123/jsep.17.4.397

Beilock, S. L. (2010). Choke: What the secrets of the brain reveal about getting it right when you have to. Free Press.

Birrer, D., & Morgan, G. (2010). Psychological skills training as a way to enhance an athlete's performance in high-intensity sports. Scandinavian Journal of Medicine & Science in Sports, 20(S2), 78–87. https://doi.org/10.1111/j.1600-0838.2010.01188.x

Gardner, F. L., & Moore, Z. E. (2007). The psychology of enhancing human performance: The mindfulness-acceptance-commitment (MAC) approach. Springer Publishing Company.

Gardner, F. L., & Moore, Z. E. (2012). Mindfulness-based and acceptance-based interventions in sport and performance contexts. Current Opinion in Psychology, 2, 73–77. https://doi.org/10.1016/j.copsyc.2015.04.010

Gross, J. J. (2015). Emotion regulation: Current status and future prospects. Psychological Inquiry, 26(1), 1–26. https://doi.org/10.1080/1047840X.2014.940781

Hayes, S. C., Strosahl, K. D., & Wilson, K. G. (2006). Acceptance and commitment therapy: An experiential approach to behavior change (2nd ed.). Guilford Press.

Kashdan, T. B., & Rottenberg, J. (2010). Psychological flexibility as a fundamental aspect of health. Clinical Psychology Review, 30(7), 865–878. https://doi.org/10.1016/j.cpr.2010.03.001

Lazarus, R. S. (2000). How emotions influence performance in competitive sports. The Sport Psychologist, 14(3), 229–252. https://doi.org/10.1123/tsp.14.3.229

Moore, Z. E. (2009). Theoretical and empirical developments of the Mindfulness-Acceptance-Commitment (MAC) approach to performance enhancement. Journal of Clinical Sport Psychology, 4(4), 291–302. https://doi.org/10.1123/jcsp.4.4.291

Vealey, R. S. (2007). Mental skills training in sport. In G. Tenenbaum & R. C. Eklund (Eds.), Handbook of sport psychology (3rd ed., pp. 287–309). Wiley.

Barnett, S. M., & Ceci, S. J. (2002). When and where do we apply what we learn? A taxonomy for far transfer. Psychological Bulletin, 128(4), 612–637. https://doi.org/10.1037/0033-2909.128.4.612

Bompa, T. O., & Buzzichelli, C. A. (2019). Periodization: Theory and methodology of training (6th ed.). Human Kinetics.

Crane, R. S., Brewer, J., Feldman, C., Kabat-Zinn, J., Santorelli, S., Williams, J. M. G., & Kuyken, W. (2019). What defines mindfulness-based programs? The warp and the weft. Psychological Medicine, 47(6), 990–999. https://doi.org/10.1017/S0033291716003317

Davidson, R. J., & Begley, S. (2012). The emotional life of your brain: How its unique patterns affect the way you think, feel, and live—and how you can change them. Penguin Books.

Kolb, B., & Gibb, R. (2011). Brain plasticity and behaviour in the developing brain. Journal of the Canadian Academy of Child and Adolescent Psychiatry, 20(4), 265–276.

Schmeichel, B. J., & Tang, D. (2015). The relationship between individual differences in self-control and neural activity. Current Directions in Psychological Science, 24(5), 354–359. https://doi.org/10.1177/0963721415593725

Tang, Y. Y., Hölzel, B. K., & Posner, M. I. (2015). The neuroscience of mindfulness meditation. Nature Reviews Neuroscience, 16(4), 213–225. https://doi.org/10.1038/nrn3916

Thomas, K., & Baker, J. (2021). Neural plasticity and skill acquisition in sport: The role of mental practice. In C. Janelle & M. Tenenbaum (Eds.), Handbook of sport psychology (4th ed., pp. 295–312). Wiley.

Beck, J. S. (2011). Cognitive behavior therapy: Basics and beyond (2nd ed.). Guilford Press.

Beilock, S. L. (2010). Choke: What the secrets of the brain reveal about getting it right when you have to. Free Press.

Conroy, D. E., & Metzler, J. N. (2004). Patterns of self-talk associated with different forms of competitive anxiety. Journal of Sport and Exercise Psychology, 26(1), 69–89. https://doi.org/10.1123/jsep.26.1.69

Cotterill, S. T. (2010). Pre-performance routines in sport: Current understanding and future directions. International Review of Sport and Exercise Psychology, 3(2), 132–153. https://doi.org/10.1080/1750984X.2010.488269

Dweck, C. S. (2006). Mindset: The new psychology of success. Random House.

Gardner, F. L., & Moore, Z. E. (2007). The psychology of enhancing human performance: The mindfulness-acceptance-commitment (MAC) approach. Springer Publishing Company.

Gross, J. J. (2015). Emotion regulation: Current status and future prospects. Psychological Inquiry, 26(1), 1–26. https://doi.org/10.1080/1047840X.2014.940781

Gucciardi, D. F., Gordon, S., & Dimmock, J. A. (2009). Advancing mental toughness research and theory using personal construct psychology. International Review of Sport and Exercise Psychology, 2(1), 54–72. https://doi.org/10.1080/17509840802705938

Hanton, S., Mellalieu, S. D., & Hall, R. (2005). Re-examining the competitive anxiety trait-state relationship. Personality and Individual Differences, 38(2), 317–329. https://doi.org/10.1016/j.paid.2004.04.005

Jones, G., Hanton, S., & Connaughton, D. (2002). What is this thing called mental toughness? An investigation of elite sport performers. Journal of Applied Sport Psychology, 14(3), 205–218. https://doi.org/10.1080/10413200290103509

Martinent, G., & Ferrand, C. (2006). A naturalistic study of the directional interpretation process of discrete emotions during high-stakes table tennis matches. Journal of Sport and Exercise Psychology, 28(4), 446–468. https://doi.org/10.1123/jsep.28.4.446

Weinberg, R. S., & Gould, D. (2019). Foundations of sport and exercise psychology (7th ed.). Human Kinetics.

Ames, C. (1992). Achievement goals and the classroom motivational climate. In J. Meece & D. Schunk (Eds.), Student perceptions in the classroom (pp. 327–348). Lawrence Erlbaum Associates.

Barnett, S. M., & Ceci, S. J. (2002). When and where do we apply what we learn? A taxonomy for far transfer. Psychological Bulletin, 128(4), 612–637. https://doi.org/10.1037/0033-2909.128.4.612

Dweck, C. S. (2006). Mindset: The new psychology of success. Random House.

Gould, D., & Voelker, D. K. (2012). Youth sport leadership development: Leveraging the sports captaincy experience. Journal of Sport Psychology in Action, 3(1), 1–14. https://doi.org/10.1080/21520704.2011.649295

Magill, R. A., & Anderson, D. I. (2017). Motor learning and control: Concepts and applications (11th ed.). McGraw-Hill Education.

Nicholls, J. G. (1989). The competitive ethos and democratic education. Harvard University Press.

Perkins, D. N., & Salomon, G. (1992). Transfer of learning. In International Encyclopedia of Education (2nd ed., Vol. 2, pp. 6452–6457). Pergamon Press.

Roberts, G. C. (2012). Motivation in sport and exercise from an achievement goal theory perspective: After 30 years, where are we?. In G. C. Roberts & D. C. Treasure (Eds.), Advances in motivation in sport and exercise (3rd ed., pp. 5–58). Human Kinetics.

Roberts, G. C., Treasure, D. C., & Conroy, D. E. (2007). Understanding the dynamics of motivation in sport and physical activity: An achievement goal interpretation. In G. Tenenbaum & R. C. Eklund (Eds.), Handbook of sport psychology (3rd ed., pp. 3–30). Wiley.

Hall, C. R., Mack, D. E., Paivio, A., & Hausenblas, H. A. (1998). Imagery use by athletes: Development of the Sport Imagery Questionnaire. International Journal of Sport Psychology, 29(1), 73–89.

Hardy, L., Jones, G., & Gould, D. (1996). Understanding psychological preparation for sport: Theory and practice of elite performers. Wiley. Jones, G. (1995). More than just a game: Research developments and issues in competitive anxiety in sport. British Journal of Psychology, 86(4), 449–478. https://doi.org/10.1111/j.2044-8295.1995.tb02565.x

Morris, T., Spittle, M., & Watt, A. P. (2005). Imagery in sport. Human Kinetics.

Sarkar, M., & Fletcher, D. (2014). Psychological resilience in sport performers: A review of stressors and protective factors. Journal of Sports Sciences, 32(15), 1419–1434. https://doi.org/10.1080/02640414.2014.901551

Theodorakis, Y., Weinberg, R., Natsis, P., Douma, I., & Kazakas, P. (2000). The effects of motivational versus instructional self-talk on improving motor performance. The Sport Psychologist, 14(3), 253–271. https://doi.org/10.1123/tsp.14.3.253

Vealey, R. S., & Greenleaf, C. A. (2010). Seeing is believing: Understanding and using imagery in sport. In J. M. Williams (Ed.), Applied sport psychology: Personal growth to peak performance (6th ed., pp. 267–299). McGraw-Hill.

Weinberg, R. S., & Gould, D. (2019). Foundations of sport and exercise psychology (7th ed.). Human Kinetics.

Baltzell, A., & Summers, J. (2017). The power of mindfulness: Mindfulness meditation training in sport (MMTS). Springer.

Birrer, D., Röthlin, P., & Morgan, G. (2012). Mindfulness to enhance athletic performance: Theoretical considerations and possible impact mechanisms. Mindfulness, 3(3), 235–246. https://doi.org/10.1007/s12671-012-0109-2

Gardner, F. L., & Moore, Z. E. (2007). The psychology of enhancing human performance: The mindfulness-acceptance-commitment (MAC) approach. Springer Publishing Company.

Gardner, F. L., & Moore, Z. E. (2012). Mindfulness and acceptance models in sport psychology: A decade of basic and applied scientific advancements. Canadian Psychology, 53(4), 309–318. https://doi.org/10.1037/a0030220

Hayes, S. C., Strosahl, K. D., & Wilson, K. G. (1999). Acceptance and commitment therapy: An experiential approach to behavior change. Guilford Press.

Jerath, R., Edry, J. W., Barnes, V. A., & Jerath, V. (2006). Physiology of long pranayamic breathing: Neural respiratory elements may provide a mechanism that explains how slow deep breathing shifts the autonomic nervous system. Medical Hypotheses, 67(3), 566–571. https://doi.org/10.1016/j.mehy.2006.02.042

Josefsson, T., Ivarsson, A., Lindwall, M., & Gustafsson, H. (2017). Mindfulness mechanisms in sports: Mediating effects of rumination and emotion regulation on sport-specific coping. Mindfulness, 8(5), 1354–1363. https://doi.org/10.1007/s12671-017-0711-4

Kabat-Zinn, J. (1990). Full catastrophe living: Using the wisdom of your body and mind to face stress, pain, and illness. Delacorte.

Moore, Z. E. (2009). Theoretical and empirical developments of the Mindfulness-Acceptance-Commitment (MAC) approach to performance enhancement. Journal of Clinical Sport Psychology, 3(4), 291–302. https://doi.org/10.1123/jcsp.3.4.291

Segal, Z. V., Williams, J. M. G., & Teasdale, J. D. (2013). Mindfulness-based cognitive therapy for depression (2nd ed.). Guilford Press.

Thompson, R. W., Kaufman, K. A., De Petrillo, L. A., Glass, C. R., & Arnkoff, D. B. (2011). One year follow-up of mindfulness-based stress reduction with cancer patients. General Hospital Psychiatry, 33(5), 426–431. https://doi.org/10.1016/j.genhosppsych.2011.05.003

Anderson, A. G., Knowles, Z., & Gilbourne, D. (2004). Reflective practice for sport psychologists: Concepts, models, practical implications, and thoughts on dissemination. The Sport Psychologist, 18(2), 188–203. https://doi.org/10.1123/tsp.18.2.188

Birrer, D., & Morgan, G. (2010). Psychological skills training as a way to enhance an athlete's performance in high-intensity sports. Scandinavian Journal of Medicine & Science in Sports, 20(S2), 78–87. https://doi.org/10.1111/j.1600-0838.2010.01188.x

Brewer, B. W., Van Raalte, J. L., & Linder, D. E. (1993). Athletic identity: Hercules' muscles or Achilles heel? International Journal of Sport Psychology, 24(2), 237–254.

Duckworth, A. L., Peterson, C., Matthews, M. D., & Kelly, D. R. (2007). Grit: Perseverance and passion for long-term goals. Journal of Personality and Social Psychology, 92(6), 1087–1101. https://doi.org/10.1037/0022-3514.92.6.1087

Gardner, F. L., & Moore, Z. E. (2007). The psychology of enhancing human performance: The mindfulness-acceptance-commitment (MAC) approach. Springer Publishing Company.

Gardner, F. L., & Moore, Z. E. (2012). Mindfulness and acceptance models in sport psychology: A decade of basic and applied scientific advancements. Canadian Psychology, 53(4), 309–318. https://doi.org/10.1037/a0030220

Gross, J. J. (2015). Emotion regulation: Current status and future prospects. Psychological Inquiry, 26(1), 1–26. https://doi.org/10.1080/1047840X.2014.940781

Gustafsson, H., Kenttä, G., Hassmén, P., & Lundqvist, C. (2011). Prevalence of burnout in adolescent competitive athletes. The Sport Psychologist, 25(4), 512–526. https://doi.org/10.1123/tsp.25.4.512

Hays, K. (2009). The psychology of performance in sport and other domains. In K. F. Hays (Ed.), Performance psychology in action: A casebook for working with athletes, performing artists, business leaders, and professionals in high-risk occupations (pp. 3–14). American Psychological Association. https://doi.org/10.1037/11876-001

Mallett, C. J., & Hanrahan, S. J. (2004). Elite athletes: Why does the "fire" burn so brightly? Psychology of Sport and Exercise, 5(2), 183–200. https://doi.org/10.1016/S1469-0292(02)00043-2

Moore, Z. E. (2009). Theoretical and empirical developments of the Mindfulness-Acceptance-Commitment (MAC) approach to performance enhancement. Journal of Clinical Sport Psychology, 3(4), 291–302. https://doi.org/10.1123/jcsp.3.4.291

Yeager, D. S., & Dweck, C. S. (2012). Mindsets that promote resilience: When students believe that personal characteristics can be developed. Educational Psychologist, 47(4), 302–314. https://doi.org/10.1080/00461520.2012.722805

Caligiore, D., Pezzulo, G., Baldassarre, G., Bostan, A. C., Strick, P. L., Doya, K., ... & Verschure, P. F. M. J. (2017). Consensus paper: Towards a systems-level view of cerebellar function: The interplay between cerebellum, basal ganglia, and cortex. The Cerebellum, 16(1), 203–229. https://doi.org/10.1007/s12311-016-0763-3

Lally, P., van Jaarsveld, C. H. M., Potts, H. W. W., & Wardle, J. (2010). How are habits formed: Modelling habit formation in the real world. European Journal of Social Psychology, 40(6), 998–1009. https://doi.org/10.1002/ejsp.674

Stanford Medicine. (2022, July 15). The science behind muscle memory. Scope. https://scopeblog.stanford.edu/2022/07/15/the-science-behind-muscle-memory/

Alvarsson, J. J., Wiens, S., & Nilsson, M. E. (2010). Stress recovery during exposure to nature sound and environmental noise. International Journal of Environmental Research and Public Health, 7(3), 1036–1046. https://doi.org/10.3390/ijerph7031036

Beck, J. S. (2011). Cognitive behavior therapy: Basics and beyond (2nd ed.). Guilford Press.

Bernstein, D. A., & Borkovec, T. D. (1973). Progressive relaxation training: A manual for the helping professions. Research Press.

Bleakley, C. M., & Davison, G. W. (2010). What is the biochemical and physiological rationale for using cold-water immersion in sports recovery? A systematic review. British Journal of Sports Medicine, 44(3), 179–187. https://doi.org/10.1136/bjsm.2009.065565

Brown, R. P., & Gerbarg, P. L. (2005). Sudarshan Kriya yogic breathing in the treatment of stress, anxiety, and depression. Journal of Alternative and Complementary Medicine, 11(4), 711–717. https://doi.org/10.1089/acm.2005.11.711

Hardy, J., Hall, C. R., & Hardy, L. (2001). Quantifying athlete self-talk. Journal of Sports Sciences, 19(9), 657–665. https://doi.org/10.1080/026404410152475806

Jacobson, E. (1938). Progressive relaxation. University of Chicago Press.

Kabat-Zinn, J. (1990). Full catastrophe living: Using the wisdom of your body and mind to face stress, pain, and illness. Delacorte.

Lundgren, J., Smith, B., & Lindström, L. (2014). Warm bath exposure and sleep quality in athletes. Journal of Sports Rehabilitation, 23(2), 120–129. https://doi.org/10.1123/jsr.2013-0004

McCorry, L. K. (2007). Physiology of the autonomic nervous system. American Journal of Pharmaceutical Education, 71(4), 78. https://doi.org/10.5688/aj710478

Sakakibara, M., Takeuchi, S., Hayano, J., & Hayano, T. (2013). Effect of slow breathing rate on cardiac parasympathetic activity in healthy adults. Journal of Physiological Anthropology, 32, Article 4. https://doi.org/10.1186/1880-6805-32-4

Taylor, A. H., & Taylor, P. (1998). Using imagery to improve sport performance. In J. L. Van Raalte & B. W. Brewer (Eds.), Exploring sport and exercise psychology (pp. 145–162). American Psychological Association.

Thoma, M. V., Ryf, S., Mohiyeddini, C., Ehlert, U., & Nater, U. M. (2013). Emotion regulation through listening to music in everyday situations. Cognition and Emotion, 27(3), 534–543. https://doi.org/10.1080/02699931.2012.740195

Wahbeh, H., Calabrese, C., & Zwickey, H. (2007). Binaural beat technology in humans: A pilot study to assess psychologic and physiologic effects. Journal of Alternative and Complementary Medicine, 13(1), 25–32. https://doi.org/10.1089/acm.2006.6196

Weil, A. (2011). Breathing: The master key to self-healing [Audio program]. Sounds True.

Abernethy, B. (2001). Attention. In R. N. Singer, H. A. Hausenblas, & C. M. Janelle (Eds.), Handbook of sport psychology (2nd ed., pp. 53–85). Wiley.

Baer, R. A. (2003). Mindfulness training as a clinical intervention: A conceptual and empirical review. Clinical Psychology: Science and Practice, 10(2), 125–143. https://doi.org/10.1093/clipsy/bpg015

Beilock, S. L., & Carr, T. H. (2001). On the fragility of skilled performance: What governs choking under pressure? Journal of Experimental Psychology: General, 130(4), 701–725. https://doi.org/10.1037/0096-3445.130.4.701

Csikszentmihalyi, M. (1990). Flow: The psychology of optimal experience. Harper & Row.

Gardner, F. L., & Moore, Z. E. (2007). The psychology of enhancing human performance: The mindfulness-acceptance-commitment (MAC) approach. Springer Publishing.

Gruzelier, J. H. (2014). EEG-neurofeedback for optimising performance. I: A review of cognitive and affective outcome in healthy participants. Neuroscience & Biobehavioral Reviews, 44, 124–141. https://doi.org/10.1016/j.neubiorev.2013.09.015

Hatfield, B. D., Haufler, A. J., Hung, T. M., & Spalding, T. W. (2004). Electroencephalographic studies of skilled psychomotor performance. Journal of Clinical Neurophysiology, 21(3), 144–156. https://doi.org/10.1097/00004691-200405000-00003

Kabat-Zinn, J. (1990). Full catastrophe living: Using the wisdom of your body and mind to face stress, pain, and illness. Delacorte.

Masters, R. S. W., & Maxwell, J. P. (2008). The theory of reinvestment. International Review of Sport and Exercise Psychology, 1(2), 160–183. https://doi.org/10.1080/17509840802287218

Moore, L. J., Vine, S. J., Wilson, M. R., & Freeman, P. (2012). The effects of challenge and threat states on performance: An examination of potential mechanisms. Psychophysiology, 49(10), 1417–1425. https://doi.org/10.1111/j.1469-8986.2012.01449.x

Thompson, M., & Thompson, L. (2003). The neurofeedback book: An introduction to basic concepts in applied psychophysiology. Association for Applied Psychophysiology and Biofeedback.

Vealey, R. S. (2007) Mental skills training in sport. In G. Tenenbaum & R. C. Eklund (Eds.), Handbook of sport psychology (3rd ed., pp. 287–309). Wiley.

Emery, M. J. (n.d.). Flow state anchors: Sports hypnosis. Retrieved from https://www.michaeljemery.com/asi-anchors-and-synesthesias-flow-state-for-athletes/

Jonov, C. (2023). Beyond the game: How achieving flow state can elevate your performance. Medium. Retrieved from https://medium.com/@colin.jonov10/beyond-the-game-how-achieving-flow-state-can-elevate-your-performance-76db69f05864

Lee, T. (2013). Overthinking can be detrimental to human performance. The Current. Retrieved from https://news.ucsb.edu/2013/013593/overthinking-can-be-detrimental-human-performance

Norsworthy, C., Gorczynski, P., & Jackson, S. A. (2017). A systematic review of flow training on flow states and performance outcomes in elite athletes. Graduate Journal of Sport, Exercise & Physical Education Research, 6, 16–28. Retrieved from https://www2.worc.ac.uk/gjseper/documents/Flow_states_and_performance_in_elite_ath letes_6_16-28.pdf

Williams, V. (2024). The neurobiology of the clutch shot: How does the brain handle pressure? Retrieved from https://www.vernonwilliamsmd.com/blog/2024/august/the-neurobiology-of-the-clutch-shot-how-does-the/

Bandura, A. (1997). Self-efficacy: The exercise of control. W.H. Freeman.

Beilock, S. L., & Carr, T. H. (2001). On the fragility of skilled performance: What governs choking under pressure? Journal of Experimental Psychology: General, 130(4), 701–725. https://doi.org/10.1037/0096-3445.130.4.701

Csikszentmihalyi, M. (1990). Flow: The psychology of optimal experience. Harper & Row.

Feltz, D. L., Short, S. E., & Sullivan, P. J. (2008). Self-efficacy in sport. Human Kinetics.

Graziano, M. S. A. (2019). Attention control and the attention schema theory of consciousness. Cognitive Neuroscience, 10(1), 1–15. https://doi.org/10.1080/17588928.2018.1488499

Harmat, L., Ørsted Andersen, F., Ullén, F., Wright, J., & Sadlo, G. (Eds.). (2016). Flow experience: Empirical research and applications. Springer.

Schmidt, R. A., & Lee, T. D. (2011). Motor control and learning: A behavioral emphasis (5th ed.). Human Kinetics.

Bandura, A. (1997). *Self-efficacy: The exercise of control*. W.H. Freeman.

Beilock, S. L., & Carr, T. H. (2001). On the fragility of skilled performance. *Journal of Experimental Psychology: General*, 130(4), 701–725.

Csikszentmihalyi, M. (1990). *Flow: The psychology of optimal experience*. Harper & Row.

Ericsson, K. A., Charness, N., Feltovich, P. J., & Hoffman, R. R. (Eds.). (2007). *The Cambridge handbook of expertise and expert performance*. Cambridge University Press.

Evans, J. S. B., & Stanovich, K. E. (2013). Dual-process theories of higher cognition. *Perspectives on Psychological Science, 8*(3), 223–241.

Graziano, M. S. (2019). *Rethinking consciousness: A scientific theory of subjective experience*. W.W. Norton.

Klein, G. (1998). *Sources of power: How people make decisions*. MIT Press.

Schmidt, R. A., & Lee, T. D. (2011). *Motor control and learning: A behavioral emphasis* (5th ed.). Human Kinetics.

Schooler, J. W. (2002). Re-representing consciousness: Dissociations between experience and meta-consciousness. *Trends in Cognitive Sciences, 6*(8), 339–344.

Swann, C., Keegan, R. J., Piggott, D., & Crust, L. (2012). A systematic review of the experience of flow in physical activity. *Psychology of Sport and Exercise, 13*(6), 807–819.

Wulf, G. (2013). Attentional focus and motor learning: A review of 15 years. *International Review of Sport and Exercise Psychology, 6*(1), 77–104.

Wulf, G., & Lewthwaite, R. (2016). Optimizing performance through intrinsic motivation and attention for learning: The OPTIMAL theory of motor learning. *Psychonomic Bulletin & Review, 23*(5), 1382–1414.

Zimmerman, B. J. (2000). Attaining self-regulation: A social cognitive perspective. In M. Boekaerts, P. R. Pintrich, & M. Zeidner (Eds.), *Handbook of self-regulation* (pp. 13–39). Academic Press.

Gleeson, B. (2018, August 7). *7 lessons from a Navy SEAL on building a culture of high performance*. Forbes. https://www.forbes.com/sites/brentgleeson/2018/08/07/7-lessons-from-a-navy-seal-on-building-a-culture-of-high-performance

Klein, G. (1998). *Sources of power: How people make decisions*. MIT Press.

Military Sphere. (n.d.). *SEAL decision-making and intuitive tactics*. Retrieved May 22, 2025, from https://www.militarysphere.com

SEAL Leadership Principles. (n.d.). *Decentralized command and mission intent*. GitBook. Retrieved May 22, 2025, from https://seal-leadership.gitbook.io

Untitled Leader. (n.d.). *The OODA Loop and adaptive leadership*. Retrieved May 22, 2025, from https://untitledleader.com

Wikipedia. (n.d.). *Recognition primed decision model*. Retrieved May 22, 2025, from https://en.wikipedia.org/wiki/Recognition-primed_decision

Zimmerman, B. J. (2000). Becoming a self-regulated learner: An overview. Theory into Practice, 41(2), 64–70. https://doi.org/10.1207/s15430421tip4102_2

Cumming, J. (2015, April 10). A sport psychologist's guide for helping athletes develop better self-awareness. Jennifer Cumming. https://jennifercumming.com/2015/04/10/a-sport-psychologists-guide-for-helping-athletes-develop-better-self-awareness/jennifercumming.com

Goleman, D. (1995). Emotional intelligence: Why it can matter more than IQ. Bantam Books.

Huffman, A. H., & Munroe-Chandler, K. J. (2021). Situation awareness in sports: A scoping review. Psychology of Sport and Exercise, 53, 101839. https://doi.org/10.1016/j.psychsport.2020.101839IRep

Laborde, S., Guillén, F., & Mosley, E. (2016). The influence of emotional intelligence on performance in competitive sports: A meta-analytic investigation. Sports Medicine, 46(9), 1203–1216. https://doi.org/10.1007/s40279-016-0491-2

NeuroTracker. (2018, March 14). Sports vision for situational awareness – Part 2. https://www.neurotrackerx.com/post/sports-vision-situational-awareness-part-2Brain Training System

Optimize Mind Performance. (2023, February 15). Self-awareness in athletes. https://optimizemindperformance.com/self-awareness-in-athletes/Trine University+2Optimize Mind Performance+2Brian Cain Peak Performance+2

Pawar, M. S. (2024). Emotional intelligence: A pivotal factor in sports performance. International Journal of Physical Education, Sports and Health, 11(5), 52–56. https://www.kheljournal.com/archives/2024/vol11issue5/PartE/11-5-52-842.pdfKhel Journal

Soles by Michelin. (2020, April 15). Self-awareness: The new edge in peak athletic performance. https://soles.michelin.com/self-awareness-the-new-edge-in-peak-athletic-performance/Soles by MICHELIN

Success Starts Within. (2023, January 10). How to improve self-awareness as an athlete. https://www.successstartswithin.com/sports-psychology-articles/emotional-intelligence-for-athletes/3-techniques-to-improve-self-awareness/successstartswithin.com

United States Center for SafeSport. (2022). The sport situational prevention approach: Implementation guide. https://uscenterforsafesport.org/wpcontent/uploads/2022/04/SSPAImplementationGuide.pdfSafeSport

Wulf, G., & Lewthwaite, R. (2016). Optimizing performance through intrinsic motivation and attention for learning: The OPTIMAL theory of motor learning. Psychonomic Bulletin & Review, 23(5), 1382–1414. https://doi.org/10.3758/s13423-015-0999-9

Cherry, K. (2023). Negative bias: Why we're hardwired for negativity. Verywell Mind. https://www.verywellmind.com/negative-bias-4589618

Collins, D., & Collins, L. (2022). The role of situational awareness in the professional judgement of sports coaches. Journal of Expertise, 5(4), 1–9. https://www.journalofexpertise.org/articles/volume5_issue4/JoE_5_4_Collins_Collins.pdf

Endsley, M. R. (1995). Toward a theory of situation awareness in dynamic systems. Human Factors, 37(1), 32–64.

Lumen Learning. (n.d.). Rational decision making vs. other types of decision making. https://courses.lumenlearning.com/wmopen-principlesofmanagement/chapter/rational-decision-making-vs-other-types-of-decision-making/

Marcora, S. M., Staiano, W., & Manning, V. (2009). Mental fatigue impairs physical performance in humans. Journal of Applied Physiology, 106(3), 857–864. https://doi.org/10.1152/japplphysiol.91324.2008

Psych Central. (2020). Emotional regulation skills: Learn how to manage your emotions. https://psychcentral.com/health/emotional-regulation

Ruhl, J. B., Salzman, J., & Clowney, D. (2020). Unpacking the complexity of environmental regulatory governance: A review of the literature. Journal of Environmental Policy & Planning, 22(2), 1–15. https://www.tandfonline.com/doi/full/10.1080/1523908X.2020.1767550

Sweller, J. (1988). Cognitive load during problem solving: Effects on learning. Cognitive Science, 12(2), 257–285. https://doi.org/10.1207/s15516709cog1202_4

Vignola, N. (2023). Rewire: Break the cycle, alter your thoughts and create lasting change. HarperCollins.

www.ingramcontent.com/pod-product-compliance
Lightning Source LLC
Chambersburg PA
CBHW060155120726
48004CB00007B/1560